**Gynaecological
and Obstetric
Pathology for
the MRCOG and
Beyond**

2nd edition

Published titles in the MRCOG and Beyond series

Forthcoming titles in the series

Gynaecological and Obstetric Pathology for the MRCOG and Beyond

Second edition

Michael Wells MD FRCPath FRCOG
Academic Unit of Pathology, University of Sheffield School of Medicine and Biomedical Sciences, Sheffield, UK

Hilary Buckley MD FRCPath
Formerly Reader in Gynaecological Pathology, Department of Pathological Sciences, University of Manchester, UK

Harold Fox MD FRCPath FRCOG
Emeritus Professor of Reproductive Pathology, Department of Pathological Sciences, University of Manchester, UK

With a chapter on cervical cytology
by John Smith FRCPath MIAC
Department of Histopathology, Royal Hallamshire Hospital, Sheffield, UK

Series Editor: Jenny Higham MD FRCOG FFFP FHEA
Consultant Gynaecologist, Professor of Medical Education and Head of Undergraduate Medicine, Faculty of Medicine, Imperial College London, UK

RCOG PRESS

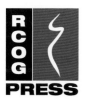

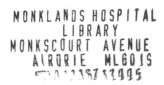
© 2009 Royal College of Obstetricians and Gynaecologists

First published 2009

Registered names: The use of registered names, trademarks, etc. in this publication does not imply, even in the absence of a specific statement, that such names are exempt from the relevant laws and regulations and therefore free for general use.

Product liability: Drugs and their doses are mentioned in this text. While every effort has been made to ensure the accuracy of the information contained within this publication, neither the authors nor the publishers can accept liability for errors or omissions. The final responsibility for delivery of the correct dose remains with the physician prescribing and administering the drug. In every individual case the respective user must check current indications and accuracy by consulting other pharmaceutical literature and following the guidelines laid down by the manufacturers of specific products and the relevant authorities in the country in which they are practising.

The rights of Michael Wells, Hilary Buckley, Harold Fox and John Smith have been asserted by them in accordance with the Copyright, Designs and Patents Act, 1988.

ISBN 978-1-904752-76-9

Published by the **RCOG Press** at the
Royal College of Obstetricians and Gynaecologists
27 Sussex Place, Regent's Park
London NW1 4RG

Registered Charity No. 213280

RCOG Press Editor: Jane Moody
Index: Liza Furnival, Medical Indexing Ltd
Design & typesetting: Karl Harrington, FiSH Books, Enfield, UK
Printed by Latimer Trend & Co. Ltd., Estover Road, Plymouth PL6 7PY, UK

Contents

Preface

Pathology – the essential science of medicine? Well, certainly a core topic and one much loved by examiners because it sorts the weaker candidates from the stronger. It is important therefore, for the serious MRCOG examination candidate to have a solid understanding of the subject where it relates to both gynaecology and obstetrics.

This textbook is a newly revised version containing concise text and many helpful colour illustrations. It is an excellent knowledge source and guide to revision, written by experts in the field. Each subject area is conveniently organised around the relevant anatomical structures. I am sure you will find this latest book in the MRCOG and Beyond Series extremely helpful.

Jenny Higham
Series Editor

Introduction to the second edition

There have been both major and minor changes in gynaecological pathology since the first edition of the book was written. Histopathologists are now much more likely to make use of immuno-histochemistry in their diagnosis, particularly of tumours, and several new pathological entities have been recognised: these have been included in this text. The manner of taking biopsies has also changed, so that endometrial biopsies, in particular, now tend to be small, superficial and fragmented and it may be impossible to assess the quality and uniformity of secretory change and, hence, to recognise an inadequate or poor response to what may have been apparently adequate hormonal stimulation. The increasing tendency to remove biopsies and even whole lesions piecemeal, as well as to collapse cysts laparoscopically, may create problems when the lesion is not, as had been anticipated, benign.

Early termination of pregnancies has made it more difficult to recognise the very early, yet equally significant, placental changes of partial and complete molar pregnancies.

The improvements in, and variety of, treatments for neoplasms has made the accurate diagnosis even more important if women are to benefit from the progress made in recent years.

We hope that this edition will be of help to gynaecologists in steering their way through the complexities of gynaecological and obstetrical histopathology.

Michael Wells
Hilary Buckley
Harold Fox

Abbreviations

AFP	α-fetoprotein
CGIN	cervical glandular intraepithelial neoplasia
CIN	cervical intraepithelial neoplasia
CIS	carcinoma in situ
ck	cytokeratin
DES	diethylstilbestrol
FIGO	International Federation of Obstetrics and Gynecology
FSH	follicle-stimulating hormone
hCG	human chorionic gonadotrophin
HIV	human immunodeficiency virus
HPV	human papillomavirus
HSV	herpes simplex virus
LH	luteinising hormone
LHRH	luteinising hormone-releasing hormone
NHSCSP	National Health Service Cervical Screening Programme
SIL	squamous intraepithelial lesions
VAIN	vaginal intraepithelial neoplasia
VIN	vulval intraepithelial neoplasia

1 The vulva

Dermatological disorders

The vulval skin is part of the body integument and is therefore subject
to all the disorders that can affect the skin elsewhere, although their
appearance may differ from that on other parts of the body; for
example, lichen planus, psoriasis or pemphigus, as well as those
conditions that affect mucous membranes. Lichen simplex, lichen
sclerosus and lichen planus merit special attention because they occur
with some frequency in the skin of the vulva. The first two disorders
were previously termed 'vulval dystrophies', a form of nomenclature
now obsolete.

LICHEN SIMPLEX

Previously classed as 'hyperplastic dystrophy', lichen simplex appears
as circumscribed areas of ill-defined, thickened red, white or brown
coloured skin, usually on the labia majora. Histologically, the
squamous epithelium is thickened and shows acanthosis, elongation of
the rete pegs, parakeratosis and hyperkeratosis with a non-specific
chronic inflammatory cell infiltrate of the dermis. Figure 1.1 shows
these epithelial changes in the absence of an inflammatory cell infiltrate of the dermis: such epithelial changes alone are simply classed as
'squamous hyperplasia' or 'squamous epithelial hyperplasia'. Lichen
simplex alone is not associated with any increased risk of vulval
carcinoma. The term lichenification is applied to similar epidermal
changes superimposed on an underlying dermatological disorder such
as eczema and may clinically mask the underlying condition.

LICHEN SCLEROSUS

Lichen sclerosus can occur in any part of the skin: (about 11% of
women have extragenital lesions) but it has a particular predilection for
the genital area. The skin lesions are papular and occur singly or in
confluent patches. Extreme pallor of the tissues and a thin fragile
epithelium with telangiectasia and gradual loss of the vulval contours

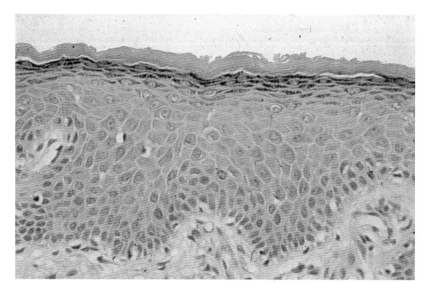

Figure 1.1. Squamous epithelial hyperplasia (lichen simplex) of the vulva: the epidermis is covered by a thick layer of keratin and the epithelium is mildly thickened (reproduced with permission from Fox and Buckley, *Atlas of Gynaecological Pathology*, published by MTP Press)

may accompany the chronic phase, with the tissues becoming parchment-like. In early lesions, bullae may form due to liquefactive degeneration of the basal layer of the epithelium and dermal oedema. In childhood, rupture of these bullae may give a false impression of sexual abuse. Histologically, the epidermis is flat and thin but may be hyperkeratotic: there is striking hyalinisation of the upper dermis and a non-specific chronic inflammatory cell infiltrate in the lower dermis (Figure 1.2). Lichen sclerosus may show secondary lichenification (Figure 1.3); this combination being previously classed as a 'mixed dystrophy'. Lichen sclerosus is not uncommonly found in association with vulval squamous carcinoma, the rate variously reported as between 4% and 96%. Although the real magnitude of this risk has not been clearly defined, it is reported that 4–6% of women with lichen sclerosus will, in time, develop squamous cell carcinoma.

LICHEN PLANUS

Lichen planus may affect the keratinised skin of the vulva, where it forms shiny, flat, polygonal violaceous papules which bear whitish

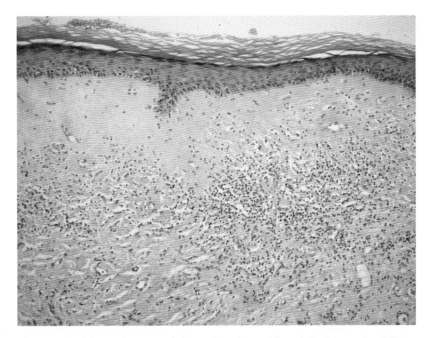

Figure 1.2. Lichen sclerosus of the vulva: the epidermis is thin and mildly hyperkeratotic and there is loss of the rete ridges; the superficial part of the underlying dermis is hyalinised, while the deeper layers are infiltrated by lymphocytes

striae, and the non-keratinised skin, where it forms reticulate, whitish lesions. Oral, vaginal and perianal lesions may coexist. The epidermis is hyperkeratotic, there is a prominent granular layer, irregular acanthosis, a sawtooth-like pattern of the rete ridges and a band-like inflammatory cell infiltrate centred on the basal layers of the epithelium (Figure 1.4). A mucocutaneous form of erosive disease is most common, affecting the inner aspects of the vulva and vagina. Lichen planus is often underdiagnosed clinically, as the late stages of the disease may, both clinically and histopathologically, resemble lichen sclerosus, presenting an atrophic, hyperkeratotic picture. The condition is associated with autoimmune disease and familial cases occur: a similar picture may occur as a reaction to some drugs and in graft versus host reaction. Women with lichen planus may develop squamous carcinoma of the vulva but the diagnosis is usually made only at the same time as the carcinoma; the frequency of this complication is, therefore, uncertain.

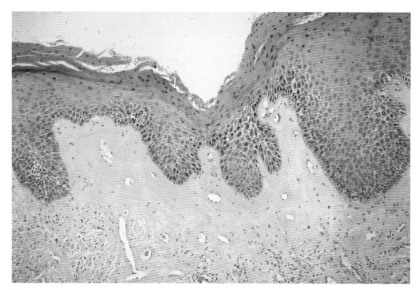

Figure 1.3. Lichen sclerosus with squamous epithelial hyperplasia and differentiated VIN: the epidermis is mildly hyperkeratotic and focally parakeratotic; the rete ridges are thickened and elongated and there is cytological atypia; the underlying superficial dermis is hyalinised

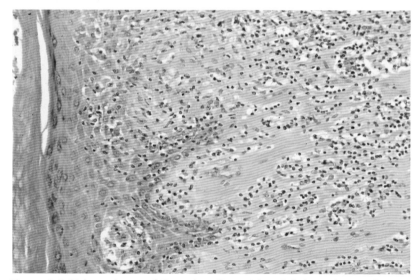

Figure 1.4. Lichen planus of the vulva: the epidermis is hyperkeratotic; there is a prominent granular layer, irregular acanthosis and a sawtooth-like pattern of the rete ridges; a band-like chronic inflammatory cell infiltrate is centred on the basal layers of the epithelium but spreads into the dermis

Inflammation of the vulva

NON-INFECTIVE VULVITIS

Non-infective inflammation of the vulva may be evoked by irritants, such as soap, scents or deodorants. Excessive washing, especially if combined with the liberal use of antiseptics, may aggravate rather than alleviate the inflammation. Incontinence of urine, a copious vaginal discharge or excessive sweating can all be irritants to vulval skin and severe vulvitis may follow exposure to radiotherapy.

The possibility that vulval inflammation may be the consequence of systemic conditions such as Crohn's disease (Figure 1.5) or ulcerative colitis should be considered.

INFECTIVE VULVITIS

Herpes virus infection

Herpetic vulvitis is not uncommon. It is acquired through sexual contact and occurs particularly in young women. The initial lesions are vesicular and may be painless. Later, the woman presents with recurrent painful ulcerative vulvitis. The histological features of the infection tend to be non-specific and diagnosis is dependent upon

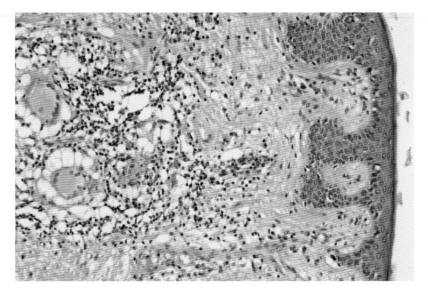

Figure 1.5. Crohn's disease of the vulva: the dermis contains a non-caseating granuloma in which two giant cells are seen surrounded by a lymphocytic infiltrate

serological studies or viral culture. The latter are important in counselling women with the condition as herpes simplex 1 (HSV-1) recurs less frequently than does HSV-2. Some women infected by the virus develop no signs or symptoms and can transmit the disease in the absence of clinical signs.

Molluscum contagiosum

Molluscum contagiosum is a common viral infection characterised by the development of discrete, asymptomatic or mildly pruritic, smooth-surfaced, pearly, skin-coloured papules or nodules. They may be single or multiple and, when mature, contain cheese-like material which can be squeezed from their centre. The papules are composed of well-demarcated, lobules of acanthotic squamous epithelium which contain viral inclusions (Figure 1.6).

Human papillomavirus

Human papillomavirus (HPV) results in the development of condylomata and vulval intraepithelial neoplasia (VIN) (see pages 8–14).

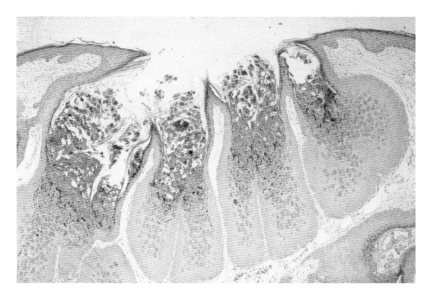

Figure 1.6. Molluscum contagiosum of the vulva: the lesion is formed by lobules of hyperplastic, acanthotic squamous epithelium which open to the surface of the skin shedding the molluscum bodies which appear darkly staining (reproduced with permission from Fox and Buckley, *Atlas of Gynaecological Pathology*, published by MTP Press)

Granuloma inguinale

This disease, possibly sexually transmitted, is caused by infection with the Gram-negative organism *Calymmatobacterium granulomatis* and is largely encountered in tropical countries. Primary lesions occur in the vulva as painful papules or nodules which break down to form a spreading ulcer with exuberant granulation tissue in its base. Healing of the lesions is by dense fibrosis which leads to extensive scarring: this may cause lymphatic obstruction with resultant vulval oedema. Histologically, there is an excessive production of non-specific granulation tissue with an infiltrate of plasma cells and histiocytes: the latter contain the rounded or rod-like Donovan bodies which are diagnostic of this disease.

Lymphogranuloma venereum

Lymphogranuloma venereum is a sexually transmitted infection with *Chlamydia trachomatis* and is most prevalent in the tropics and sub-tropics. The primary lesion is a self-healing vulval papule or shallow ulcer which is later followed by a suppurative inguinal lymphadenitis: the large painful nodes become matted together and liquefy to form fluctuant buboes which drain through the skin via indolent sinuses. In a proportion of cases, the primary lesions do not heal and progress to a chronic spreading destructive ulceration, which may involve the vulva, vagina and rectum, leading eventually to vaginal and rectal stenoses. Histologically, characteristic features are present only in the lymph nodes where stellate abscesses are seen.

Syphilis

The vulva is a site of predilection for the primary lesion of syphilis, the chancre, which appears as a painless, hard, brownish-red nodule, often with surface erosion. This heals spontaneously after a few weeks. The typical silvery-grey snail-track ulcers of the secondary stage of syphilis can occur on the vulva, whereas elevated moist plaques, known as condylomata lata, may involve not only the vulva in secondary syphilis but also the adjacent perineum, perianal region and upper thighs.

Chancroid

Chancroid is a sexually-transmitted acute infection by *Haemophilus ducrei*. The primary lesions develop on the labia as painful nodules, often multiple, which break down to form small erosions. These tend to coalesce to form large ragged irregular ulcers with an excavated margin. The infection commonly spreads to the inguinal nodes to produce a painful lymphadenitis which may evolve into fluctuant masses that discharge through the skin. The histological appearances are of non-specific granulation tissue.

Candida

Infection of the vulva by *Candida albicans* is usually associated with infection in the vagina. It presents with soreness and itching and can be diagnosed by means of a scraping or swab, although in practice it is often diagnosed clinically (Figure 1.7).

CONDYLOMA ACUMINATUM

Condyloma acuminatum lesions, also known as venereal or genital warts, occur most commonly in young women and their incidence has been increasing in recent years. Lesions may be a particular problem in women who are immunosuppressed. The condylomata typically occur along the edges of the labia minora, between the labia minora and majora, around the introitus and on the perineal and perianal skin. They are usually multiple and often confluent. Macroscopically, they appear as papillary or verrucous lesions which may be pedunculated or sessile. Histologically (Figure 1.8), complex fibrovascular cores are covered by acanthotic squamous epithelium which shows parakeratosis and, often, hyperkeratosis. Multinucleation, premature individual cell keratini-

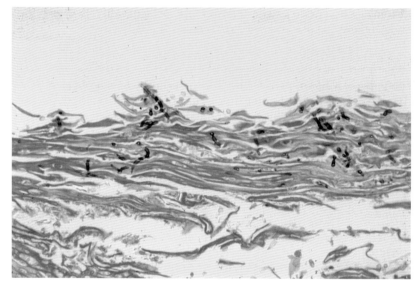

Figure 1.7. Candidal infection of the vulva: fine, darkly staining fungal hyphae can be seen lying within the hyperkeratotic layer of the epidermis (Silver stain)

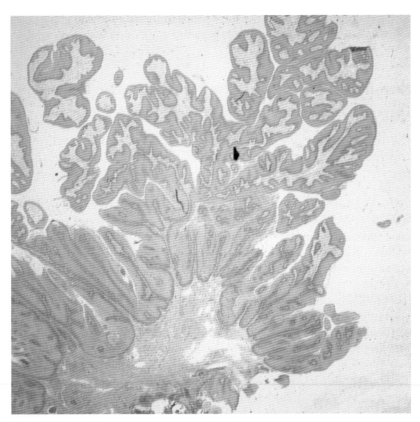

Figure 1.8. Condyloma acuminatum: fine fibrovascular cores are covered by acanthotic squamous epithelium which is mildly hyperkeratotic

sation and koilocytosis are usually present. Koilocytosis is a viral cytopathic effect characterised by nuclear irregularities and cytoplasmic vacuolation.

Condylomata acuminata are caused by infection with HPV types 6 or 11: the infection is usually sexually transmitted but is occasionally acquired in children as a result of non-sexual contact. They do not show any tendency to undergo neoplastic change but are, nevertheless, associated with an increased incidence of concomitant VIN and cervical intraepithelial neoplasia (CIN).

Sometimes vulval skin that appears normal to naked-eye examination may have histological features similar to those seen in the epithelium covering a condyloma acuminatum. Such lesions are called flat condylomata or subclinical HPV infection and have their counterparts on the cervix. Their significance lies in the fact that they, too, may be associated with VIN but may escape detection during ordinary clinical examination.

Non-invasive, intraepithelial neoplastic lesions

VULVAL INTRAEPITHELIAL NEOPLASIA

The term VIN encompasses and replaces those conditions previously known as Bowen's disease, Bowenoid papulosis, erythroplasia of Queyrat, dysplasia, squamous carcinoma in situ and dystrophy with atypia.

The incidence of VIN appears to have increased markedly during the last 35 years, particularly in younger women. In view of the high incidence of associated CIN, it is not surprising that many of the epidemiological factors operative for CIN, such as early onset of sexual activity, oral contraceptive use and multiple sexual partners, are also associated with VIN. Woman with immune deficiency are at particular risk of all manifestations of HPV infection.

A clear association between VIN and HPV types 16 and 18 infection has been abundantly demonstrated. A significant proportion of cases of VIN are, however, negative for HPV and it is now clear that there are two types of VIN. One, associated with HPV infection, occurs predominantly but by no means solely in younger women (mean age at diagnosis 49 years) and tends to be a multicentric and multifocal disease, while the second, which is non-HPV-associated, is usually found in older women (mean age at diagnosis 60 years) and is commonly unifocal and unicentric. There also appears to be a clear correlation between VIN and cigarette smoking in younger women.

The most common complaint of women with VIN 3 is pruritus. About one-third will have noticed an abnormality of the vulval skin and a substantial proportion are asymptomatic. The lesion is detected incidentally during the investigation or treatment of a woman with vulval condylomata, CIN or abnormal cervical cytology by means of colposcopy, which should always include colposcopic evaluation of the vagina and vulva. As many as two-thirds of women with VIN 3 have evidence of HPV-associated disease in other sites.

VIN may be discrete and sharply localised but can involve the entire vulva, the perineum and perianal areas; the most frequent site for a discrete lesion is the labium minus.

The gross appearances are extremely variable: the lesions may be white, dull grey, red, brown, variegated red and white or darkly pigmented and they may be flat, granular or warty.

Histologically, VIN may be undifferentiated or differentiated, the former tending to occur in younger women and being frequently associated with both HPV infection and smoking and the latter occurring more commonly in older women and usually not associated with HPV infection.

THE TWO BASIC PATTERNS OF UNDIFFERENTIATED, HPV-ASSOCIATED VIN

In **basaloid** VIN (Figure 1.9), cells of basal or parabasal type extend into the upper layers of the epidermis.

In **Bowenoid** (or 'warty') VIN (Figure 1.10), premature cellular maturation occurs, often in association with epithelial multinucleation, corps ronds and koilocytosis.

Common to both forms of VIN is the presence of often abnormal mitotic figures, above the basal layers of the epithelium, cellular and nuclear pleomorphism, a high nucleocytoplasmic ratio, irregular clumping of nuclear chromatin and, in many cases, either parakeratosis or hyperkeratosis. It is not uncommon in both forms of VIN for pigmentary incontinence to occur and for the underlying dermis to contain large numbers of melanin-laden macrophages. These are responsible for the pigmentation, which is sometimes macroscopically apparent (Figure 1.11). The two forms of undifferentiated VIN may exist together in the same patient and are not mutually exclusive.

In differentiated VIN, the epithelium shows little or no atypia above the basal or parabasal layers but large, apparently prematurely matured, eosinophilic keratinocytes with abnormal nuclei are present in the basal layers and such cells or intraepithelial pearls are also present in the rete ridges. It is usual to grade undifferentiated VIN and the World Health Organization grading system is widely used (Table 1.1).

Using this system, grading of a basaloid VIN is relatively easy but the grading of an overtly HPV-associated VIN is often difficult and sometimes impossible. A differentiated VIN cannot be graded but should probably be regarded, for clinical purposes, as VIN 3. The diagnosis of VIN1 tends, however, to be poorly reproducible while the risk of this lesion evolving into an invasive carcinoma is almost certainly extremely low and the disease may be self-limiting. Because of this there is an increasing tendency to eliminate VIN1 as a diagnostic entity and to combine VIN2 and VIN3 into the single category of VIN.

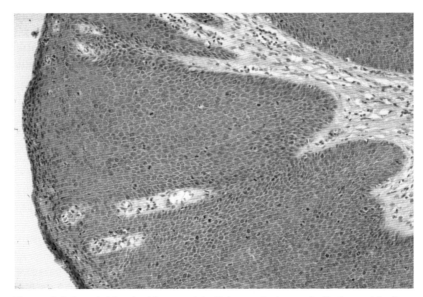

Figure 1.9. Basaloid vulval intraepithelial neoplasia grade 3: the epithelium is occupied throughout its thickness by cells resembling those of the normal basal layer

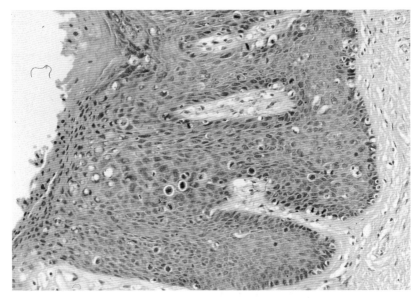

Figure 1.10. 'Bowenoid' vulval intraepithelial neoplasia grade 3: the cellular atypia is characterised by the presence of koilocytes, corps ronds and frequent mitoses; the surface may be hyperkeratotic or parakeratotic, or both, as in this case

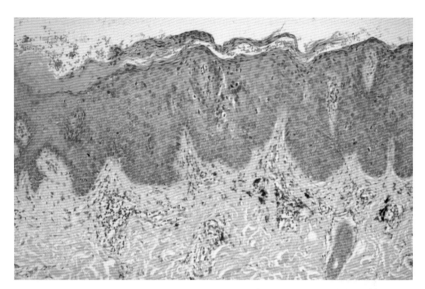

Figure 1.11. Pigmentary incontinence in vulval intraepithelial neoplasia (VIN): the accumulation of melanin shed from the epidermis and retained in macrophages in the dermis may cause the VIN to appear pigmented; it is important to distinguish such lesions from melanocytic lesions

Table 1.1 World Health Organization grading system for grading undifferentiated VIN	
Grade	**Definition**
1	Nuclear abnormalities are present in all layers of the epithelium but a lack of both stratification and cytoplasmic differentiation are limited to the lower third of the epithelium
2	Nuclear abnormalities are present in all layers of the epithelium but a failure of stratification and cytoplasmic maturation extends into the middle third of the epithelium
3	Nuclear abnormalities are present throughout the epithelium but there may be some degree of cytoplasmic maturation in the upper third of the epithelium

There is no doubt that VIN 3 can progress to an invasive squamous cell carcinoma and carcinoma may be detected unexpectedly when VIN has been resected. The potential for progression of VIN 3 to an invasive carcinoma, particularly the HPV-associated type in younger women, has generally been thought to be low and is usually estimated to be no more than 3–4%. The risk of invasion is not, however, consistently low and it is possible that it has been seriously underestimated in the past, particularly in elderly women, in whom progression to an invasive lesion can occur in up to 19% of VIN cases.

PAGET'S DISEASE

Vulval Paget's disease is rare and occurs most commonly in postmenopausal women, in whom it presents as often multiple, poorly demarcated, erythematous areas in any part of the vulval skin. Histologically (Figure 1.12), there are large, round or oval cells with pale cytoplasm, lying singly or in nests within the epidermis: glandular differentiation is seen in a few cases. The Paget cells stain positively for low molecular weight cytokeratins (Figure 1.13), contain mucus and are periodic acid Schiff-positive after diastase digestion, characteristics which help to differentiate them from melanocytes.

Paget's disease of the vulva can arise in two ways. In a minority of cases there is a subjacent adnexal adenocarcinoma or anorectal carcinoma, the Paget cells representing an extension or metastasis from this to the epidermis. In most women, however, there is no associated adenocarcinoma and the Paget cells develop in situ from pluripotential undifferentiated cells in the basal layers of the vulval epithelium. Under these circumstances, the Paget cells represent an intraepithelial adenocarcinoma, which can occasionally progress to an invasive lesion.

Non-neoplastic cysts

Cysts forming in developmental remnants are those of mesonephric duct or peritoneal origin. The former develop in the lateral part of the labium majus and are lined by a cuboidal epithelium; they contain clear serous fluid. Cysts of peritoneal origin develop in the fragment of peritoneum which may accompany the round ligament into the vulva; the resulting cyst is lined by mesothelium, contains clear watery fluid, and lies in the upper part of the labium majus.

Epidermoid cysts, which are lined by stratified squamous epithelium and contain laminated keratinous debris, occur most commonly in the labia majora, where they probably develop in the ducts of sebaceous glands, and in the perineal area, where they occur in obstetric scars.

Obstruction of one of the minor mucus-secreting glands in the vestibule leads to the formation of a mucous cyst lined by a cubo-columnar, mucin-secreting epithelium. The largest and only individually named gland of this type is Bartholin's gland. Cysts developing in the

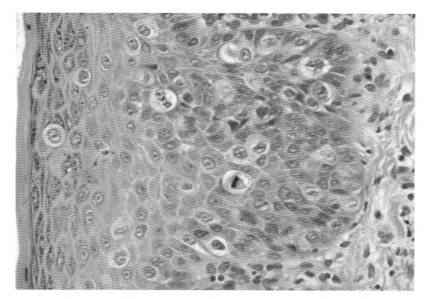

Figure 1.12. Paget's disease of the vulva: within the epidermis, most conspicuously in the deeper half, there are groups of large Paget cells with pale cytoplasm, atypical nuclei and occasional mitotic figures (reproduced with permission from Tindall, Baldwin, Buckley and Turner, 1997, published by Mosby-Wolfe)

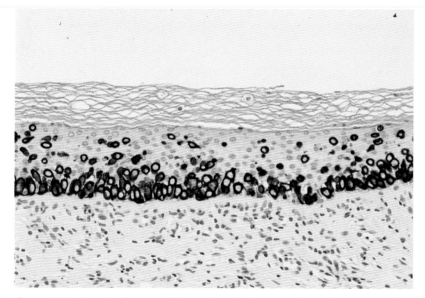

Figure 1.13. Paget's disease of the vulva: the Paget cells are here stained with an antibody to low molecular weight cytokeratin (CAM 5.2)

gland duct lie in the posterolateral part of the labium majus and most commonly follow obstruction due to post-inflammatory fibrosis or inspissation of secretions. The cysts are lined by squamous, transitional or columnar epithelium (Figure 1.14), depending upon the level at which the obstruction occurred.

Benign tumours

Benign epithelial tumours of the vulva are more common than benign mesenchymal neoplasms, which are rare.

Epithelial tumours develop from the epidermis and the skin appendages. The most common of the epidermal tumours are squamous papilloma, fibroepitheliomatous polyp, basal cell papilloma and keratoacanthoma. Occasionally, intradermal or compound naevi are seen. Squamous papillomas and fibroepitheliomatous polyps (skin tags) are of similar appearance and consist of vascular connective tissue covered by mildly acanthotic and hyperkeratotic squamous epithelium; they are most common in the middle aged and elderly.

Basal cell papillomas (seborrhoeic keratoses) are small, exophytic, pigmented lesions which appear to be stuck on the skin. They are composed of sheets of small, regular cells resembling the normal basal cells of the epidermis and in many there are keratin-containing cysts.

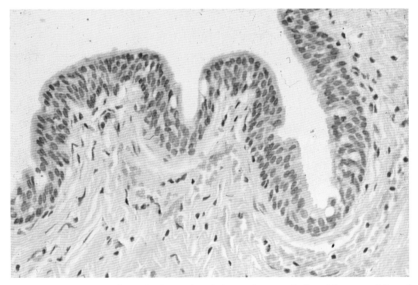

Figure 1.14. A cyst of Bartholin's gland duct: the cyst is lined by transitional epithelium covered by mucus-secreting columnar epithelium

Keratoacanthomas are rapidly growing, self-limiting neoplasms which may be of viral origin. They consist of lobules of well-differentiated squamous cell masses arranged around a central keratin-plugged crater.

Tumours may also develop from the sweat glands, one of the most common of these in the vulva being the papillary hidradenoma. Hidradenomas are small, painless subcutaneous swellings, usually on the labia majora, and have a complex tubular, acinar and papillary histological pattern (Figure 1.15).

Vulval mesenchymal tumours have a tendency to become pedunculated. Fibromas, leiomyomas, lipomas, haemangiomas, neurofibromas, neurilemmomas and granular cell tumours also occur.

Malignant tumours

INVASIVE SQUAMOUS CELL CARCINOMA

Squamous cell carcinoma accounts for 80–90% of malignant vulval neoplasms and for about 3–4% of gynaecological cancers. While squamous carcinoma occurs most commonly in women over the age of 60 years, the incidence in younger women is increasing and some reports suggest that 60% of cases now occur in women less than 60 years of age. The common presenting complaints are of a vulval lump, pruritus, discharge, bleeding and pain.

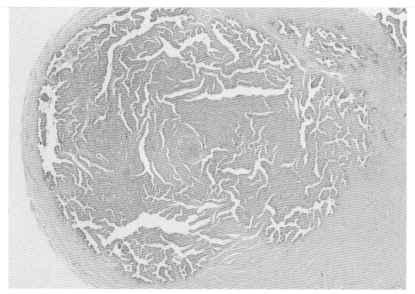

Figure 1.15. A hidradenoma of the vulva: within the dermis there is a well-circumscribed nodule composed of tightly packed glandular acini

The majority of squamous carcinomas (70%) develop on the labia, most commonly the labia majora; the second most common site is the clitoris. Over 50% of the tumours are ulcerated while about 33% are papillary and about 10% are plaque-like.

In recent years, squamous cell carcinomas of the vulva have been subdivided into three separate categories, which differ from each other not only in their histological appearances but also in their relationship to patient age, association with HPV infection and origin from pre-existing VIN.

THREE CATEGORIES OF SQUAMOUS CELL CARCINOMAS

1 Typical keratinising squamous cell carcinoma
2 Basaloid carcinoma
3 Warty carcinoma

Typical keratinising squamous cell carcinomas (Figure 1.16) account for about 65% of cases. They occur predominantly in women over 65 years of age and are infrequently associated with HPV infection. The adjacent non-involved epithelium usually shows squamous hyperplasia or lichen sclerosus and VIN is relatively rarely seen. When present, it tends to be of the differentiated type. Most are well-

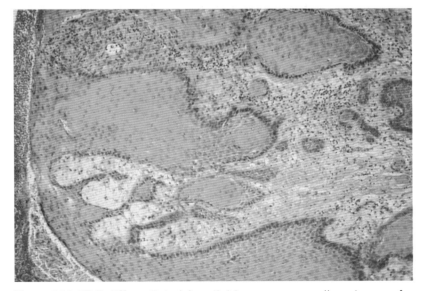

Figure 1.16. Well-differentiated, keratinising squamous cell carcinoma of the vulva; note the characteristic epithelial pearls

differentiated squamous cell carcinomas and form rounded nests of mature squamous cells with keratin pearls, with tongues of cells extending down into the dermis and subcutaneous tissues. Poorly differentiated forms of squamous carcinoma may show little evidence of keratinisation and may consist of spindle shaped cells.

Basaloid carcinomas form about 28% of invasive neoplasms, are frequently associated with HPV strains 16 and 18 and occur in relatively young women, usually below the age of 60 years. The adjacent non-involved epithelium commonly shows a basaloid type of VIN 3. The tumours are formed of masses, nests, clusters or cords of basal-type cells with scanty cytoplasm and a high nucleocytoplasmic ratio.

Warty carcinomas constitute approximately 7% of invasive carcinomas, occur in younger women (mean age 49 years at diagnosis) and are associated with oncogenic HPV infection: the adjacent uninvolved epithelium usually shows an HPV-associated (Bowenoid) VIN 3. These tumours are formed of irregularly-shaped nests of epithelium in which there is a variable degree of nuclear pleomorphism and cytological atypia with multinucleated cells and koilocytes. Approximately 40% of women with basaloid and warty carcinomas also have CIN. In contrast, only 2% of women with typical squamous carcinomas have cervical neoplasia.

Squamous carcinomas spread directly to adjacent tissues, by the lymphatics to the inguinal, femoral and pelvic nodes and, rarely, late in the course of the disease, by the bloodstream to the lungs, liver and bones. Nearly 30% of women have inguinal nodal metastases at the time of initial diagnosis and 10–20% have pelvic node metastases.

The older FIGO staging system using only clinical data was highly inaccurate, particularly with respect to the presence or absence of groin lymph node metastases, and has been replaced by a combined clinical and surgical staging system (Table 1.2). It is now accepted that the presence of groin nodal metastases must be pathologically confirmed. The overall 5-year survival rate for women with vulval carcinoma is now about 75%. For women with no nodal metastases, the survival rate is 90–100% while for those with inguinal spread the survival rate is 30–70%, falling to less than 25% if pelvic nodes are involved. The single most important factor governing prognosis is the absence or otherwise of nodal spread and, while various tumour-associated factors, such as tumour diameter, tumour thickness, tumour differentiation, tumour grade, the presence of vascular space invasion and pattern of tumour growth appear to be of prognostic value, it is probable that these are largely indicative of the risk of, and are subordinate to, nodal metastases. Sentinel lymph node biopsy may, in the future, reduce the need for radical lymphadenectomy.

Table 1.2 Combined clinical and pathological staging of vulval carcinoma (FIGO 1995)

Stage	Definition
I	Tumour confined to the vulva, 2 cm or less in diameter, no metastases in the groin nodes
Ia	depth of invasion not exceeding 1 mm (calculated from the dermo-epidermal junction of the nearest, most superficial dermal papilla)
Ib	all others
II	Tumour confined to the vulva, more than 2 cm in diameter, no metastases in the groin nodes
III	Tumour of any size with adjacent spread to the vagina, urethra and/or perineum and/or anus and/or unilateral pathologically confirmed groin lymph node metastases
IVa	Tumour of any size infiltrating the bladder mucosa and/or rectal mucosa, including the upper part of the urethral mucosa, and/or fixed to the bone and/or pathologically confirmed bilateral groin lymph node metastases
IVb	Distant metastases and/or pathologically confirmed pelvic lymph node metastases

MICROINVASIVE SQUAMOUS CELL CARCINOMA

Attempts to define a microinvasive carcinoma of the vulva which might be treated relatively conservatively in a manner similar to that of cervical microinvasive carcinoma have met with variable success. Only when invasion is less than 1 mm from the epithelial stromal junction of the adjacent, most superficial dermal papilla to the deepest point of invasion can the lesion be treated conservatively (Figure 1.17) because lymph node metastases are unlikely. Any tumour in which there is a confluent growth pattern or even a suspicion of vascular involvement cannot be regarded as minimally invasive, no matter how small or superficial.

VERRUCOUS CARCINOMA

Verrucous carcinoma is a rare but distinctive variant of a squamous cell carcinoma which may be associated with HPV type 6 in particular but in some cases there is no precursor lesion. Giant condyloma is considered by some to be synonymous with verrucous carcinoma. The tumour presents, usually in the postmenopausal years, as a slowly-growing,

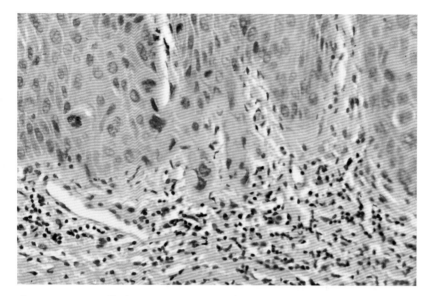

Figure 1.17. So-called 'microinvasive' squamous cell carcinoma: two buds of superficial squamous cell carcinoma show early stromal invasion of the dermis from an epithelium in which there are features of vulval intraepithelial neoplasia grade 3

bulky, fungating, cauliflower-like mass. Histologically, these neoplasms have a remarkably bland appearance with little evidence of cellular atypia or mitotic activity. The base of the tumour is well circumscribed with bulbous rete ridges which appear to be compressing, rather than invading, the underlying tissues. Histologically, a biopsy may be mistaken for a condyloma acuminatum and it is important that the histopathologist is provided with the details of the clinical features.

These tumours rarely metastasise to lymph nodes but tend to show a relentless local invasiveness and commonly recur after excision. Treatment is by surgery as they respond to radiotherapy by assuming an even more aggressive stance.

MALIGNANT MELANOMA

Between 3% and 5% of malignant melanomas in women occur in the vulval skin. Such neoplasms constitute between 4% and 5% of all malignant vulval tumours and occur predominantly in the sixth decade of life. The labia majora, labia minora and clitoris are involved with about equal frequency and the melanoma may be of the superficial spreading, nodular or acral lentiginous type (Figure 1.18).

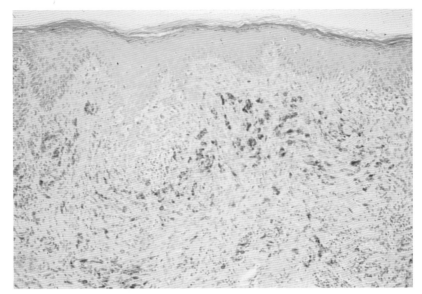

Figure 1.18. Malignant melanoma: the dermis is infiltrated by pigmented melanoma cells; although this is quite a deep lesion, it is not unusual for vulval melanomas to present late

The overall 5-year survival rate for women with a malignant melanoma of the vulva is about 30–40%. The tumour tends to present relatively late, to spread early to the inguinal nodes and to be widely disseminated via the bloodstream. The prognosis for tumours still localised to the vulva depends upon the thickness of the neoplasm and its depth of invasion.

Other pigmented lesions of the vulva also occur and must be differentiated from malignant melanoma. These include Bowenoid VIN with pigmentary incontinence (Figure 1.11), basal cell papilloma, lentigo, intradermal, junctional and compound naevi and basal cell carcinoma.

BASAL CELL CARCINOMA

Basal cell carcinomas account for only 2–10% of vulval neoplasms and tend to develop on the labia majora in the elderly. The tumours often present as a polypoidal or plaque-like ulcerated mass and tend to be multifocal. The vulval tumours are of a similar histological pattern and clinical behaviour to those encountered elsewhere in the body. About 20% recur locally after excision, usually as a result of incomplete removal, but lymph node metastases are exceptional (Figure 1.19).

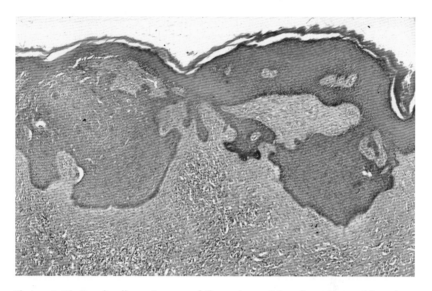

Figure 1.19. Basal cell carcinoma of the vulva: arising from the epidermis there are multiple, irregular cellular proliferations which are typical of basal cell carcinoma

ADENOCARCINOMA

Adenocarcinomas are rare primary neoplasms of the vulva and are most likely to develop from skin adnexa, Bartholin's gland, embryonic duct remnants, endometriotic foci or ectopic breast tissue. The possibility that an adenocarcinoma found in the vulva is actually a metastatic tumour should always be considered (see below).

MALIGNANT ADNEXAL (SKIN APPENDAGE) NEOPLASMS

These rare tumours present a wide variety of histological patterns and develop from sweat glands and sebaceous glands. Adenocarcinomas of tubular, myxoid and spindle cell form, apocrine adenocarcinomas resembling breast carcinoma, adenosquamous carcinomas, mucoid carcinomas and sebaceous carcinomas are all recognised. Local recurrence and metastasis are common.

CARCINOMA OF BARTHOLIN'S GLAND

Carcinomas of Bartholin's gland are rare and tend to occur at a peak age of about 50 years. The tumour usually presents as a vulval nodule or mass which tends eventually to ulcerate through the overlying skin. The presence of a Bartholin's gland abscess in an older women should alert the clinician to the possibility of an underlying carcinoma. Most of the neoplasms are either adenocarcinomas or squamous cell carcinomas (the latter probably arising from foci of metaplastic squamous epithelium within the ducts) but about 15% are adenoid cystic carcinomas.

Adenocarcinomas and squamous cell carcinomas tend to avail themselves of the rich lymphatic drainage of Bartholin's gland and metastasise first to the inguinal nodes then to the deep pelvic nodes, the 5-year survival rate for women with these tumours being only about 30%. Adenoid cystic adenocarcinomas show less tendency to metastasise but are locally highly aggressive, invading extensively and recurring with considerable frequency.

URETHRAL CARCINOMA

Urethral carcinoma, although rare, is more common in women than men, affecting particularly elderly women. Tumours of the distal urethra are more common than those in the proximal, or posterior, urethra.

In the distal urethra, tumours are usually squamous or transitional, whereas in the proximal urethra adenocarcinomas also occur. Women in whom disease is limited to the distal urethra do well but tumours involving the whole urethra or only its proximal portion have a poor prognosis because in many such cases metastases have already occurred at the time of diagnosis.

MALIGNANT SOFT TISSUE TUMOURS

Malignant soft tissue tumours of the vulva are uncommon but leiomyosarcomas are the least infrequent. Aggressive angiomyxoma is an uncommon lesion which presents as a painless expanding mass in the vulva of women usually under the age of 40 years. Histologically, it has a remarkably bland appearance yet infiltrates the soft tissues of the vulva, paravaginal areas and extends to the pelvic tissues (Figure 1.20), this latter characteristic accounting for the frequent recurrence after surgical removal.

METASTATIC CARCINOMAS

The possibility that rare tumours of the vulva, such as adenocarcinoma, might be metastatic should always be borne in mind, as the vulva is not an uncommon site of metastases from the cervix, endometrium, vagina, ovary, urethra, kidney, breast, rectum and lung (Figure 1.21).

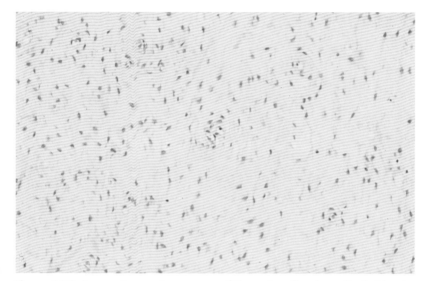

Figure 1.20. Aggressive angiomyxoma of the vulva: the deceptively bland lesion is composed of regular spindle-shaped cells set in a myxoid stroma in which there are small blood vessels

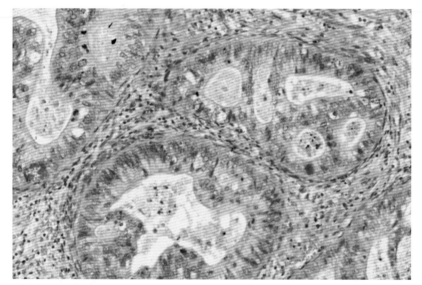

Figure 1.21. Metastatic intestinal adenocarcinoma: the history of previous large intestinal carcinoma should raise the suspicion of metastatic disease, although primary carcinomas of this type may occur rarely in the vulva

2 The vagina

Vaginal inflammation

NON-INFECTIVE INFLAMMATION

Non-infective vaginal inflammation may complicate trauma, surgery, irradiation, the introduction of foreign bodies, the application of chemical substances or the wearing of a pessary. These factors are more likely to cause inflammatory changes at times of estrogen deficiency, for example after the menopause.

INFECTIVE INFLAMMATION

Most vaginal infections are sexually transmitted but it is far from certain how the infecting organisms become established in the vagina and overcome the dual threats posed by the normal vaginal flora and the acidity of vaginal fluids. It is probable that changes in estrogen or progesterone levels are an important factor in the establishment of an infection, in so far as estrogen deficiency or progesterone excess will result in diminished epithelial growth, a reduction in the supply of glycogen and restriction of the ability of lactobacilli to flourish, thus allowing invading organisms to gain ascendancy.

Bacterial vaginosis

The sexually transmitted Gram-negative bacillus, *Gardnerella vaginalis*, either acting singly or in combination with anaerobic organisms, is now recognised to be the cause of the vast majority of cases previously designated as 'non-specific vaginitis'. Bacterial vaginosis is associated with a thin, watery, highly malodorous vaginal discharge but the organism is only a surface parasite and does not invade the vaginal tissues or evoke any inflammatory reaction.

Candidiasis

Candida albicans may exist in the vagina without causing any signs or symptoms. The fungal organism can, however, change from a saprophyte to a pathogen if the host is immunosuppressed or if growth of the normal vaginal flora is inhibited by, for example, the use of broad-spectrum antibiotics. Such a change also often occurs in pregnancy when high estrogen levels may be associated with increased cellular glycogen concentration. Once allowed to proliferate freely, *C. albicans* penetrates focally into the vaginal epithelium and initiates a vaginitis. The vaginal epithelium is congested and whitish plaques may be seen on the vaginal surface; these are easily removed to expose a reddened 'raw' area.

Trichomoniasis

The unicellular protozoal parasite *Trichomonas vaginalis* is one of the most common causes of vaginitis. The parasite is usually sexually transmitted but can on occasion be transmitted via fomites. The acute stage of the infection is characterised by a frothy vaginal discharge and the vaginal skin has a reddish granular appearance. Histologically, congestion, oedema and a lymphoplasmocytic infiltrate of the subepithelial papillae are characteristic features. The inflammatory infiltrate may extend into the epithelium and form small intraepithelial abscesses (see Figure 3.8 on page 43). The infection may progress into a chronic state, although some women become symptomless carriers of the parasite.

Gonorrhoea

The thick, squamous epithelium of the adult vagina is resistant to gonococcal infection. In children, however, the thin epithelium is permeable to the organism, which can produce a vaginitis.

Syphilis

The vagina is an uncommon site for a chancre but the mucosal 'snail-track' ulcers and condylomata lata of secondary syphilis can affect the lower vagina. Tertiary-stage lesions are only rarely encountered in the vagina.

Vaginal adenosis

Vaginal adenosis, which is usually asymptomatic but is occasionally associated with a vaginal discharge, is characterised by the presence of glandular structures in the lamina propria of the vagina (Figure 2.1), with some opening on to the vaginal surface. The glands are most commonly lined by a mucinous, endocervical-type epithelium but may have a lining of endometrial or tubal type. The glands have a marked tendency to undergo squamous metaplasia and, in older women, may eventually be completely replaced by squamous tissue.

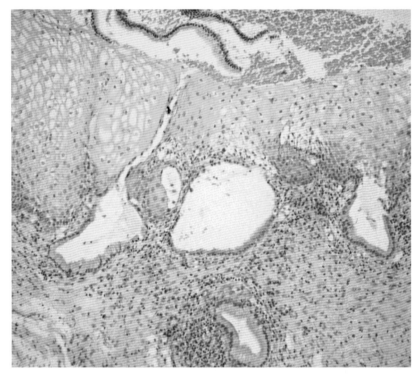

Figure 2.1. The epithelium lining the vagina is of normal stratified squamous type but in the underlying stroma there are glands lined by mucus-secreting epithelium of endocervical type

Vaginal adenosis is thought to be caused by sequestration of müllerian elements during vaginal embryogenesis and is indicative of a disturbance in the orderly replacement of the lower parts of the müllerian ducts by the squamous epithelium of the urogenital sinus. The condition may occur spontaneously but was particularly common in women who were exposed prenatally to diethylstilbestrol (DES), being found in 70% of girls exposed to DES during the first 8 weeks of fetal life.

Vaginal adenosis is not, in itself, of any major clinical importance but it is of considerable significance as a precursor of clear-cell adenocarcinoma of the vagina (see below).

Vaginal intraepithelial neoplasia

Vaginal intraepithelial neoplasia (VAIN) has been studied much less intensively than have VIN and CIN and its natural history is poorly understood. The lesion is often multifocal, usually asymptomatic and is discovered only on routine examination, when it is seen either as an area of increased vascularity or as a whitish patch. A high proportion of women with VAIN have been previously treated for either intraepithelial or invasive neoplasia of the cervix and it is thought that the aetiological factors for VAIN are similar to those for CIN (see page 46).

The histological appearances of VAIN are similar to those of both VIN and CIN and include delayed maturation of the squamous cells, disturbance in polarity, an increased nucleocytoplasmic ratio, nuclear pleomorphism, the finding of mitotic figures above the basal layers and the presence of abnormal mitotic figures. Classification of VAIN is shown in Table 2.1.

Table 2.1 Classification of VAIN lesions	
Class	Definition
1	Nuclear abnormalities are present in all layers of the epithelium but a lack of both stratification and cytoplasmic differentiation are limited to the lower third of the epithelium
2	Nuclear abnormalities are present in all layers of the epithelium but a failure of stratification and cytoplasmic maturation extends into the middle third of the epithelium
3	Nuclear abnormalities are present throughout the epithelium but there may be some cytoplasmic maturation in the upper third of the epithelium

VAIN is widely regarded as a precursor of an invasive squamous cell carcinoma of the vagina but neither its invasive potential nor its quantitative importance as a precursor of malignant vaginal neoplasia have been adequately defined.

Vaginal neoplasms

Malignant neoplasms of the vagina are rare, accounting for only about 1% of cancers of the female genital tract. A malignant neoplasm in the vagina is more likely to be a metastasis from sites such as the colon (Figure 2.2), endometrium or kidney than a primary vaginal tumour.

SQUAMOUS CARCINOMA

Neoplasms of this type account for 95% of malignant vaginal tumours

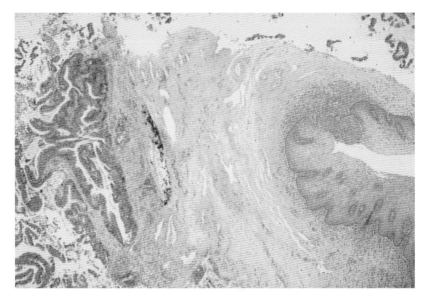

Figure 2.2. Colonic carcinoma growing into the vagina: the vaginal mucosa, to the right, is composed of normal stratified squamous epithelium and in the deep tissues, to the left, there is well-differentiated adenocarcinoma of intestinal type

and occur predominantly in women in their sixth or seventh decades. Squamous carcinomas develop most commonly in the posterior wall of the upper third of the vagina, usually present as an exophytic fungating mass and are often moderately differentiated. The tumour invades, at a relatively early stage, adjacent structures such as the cervix, perivaginal tissues, bladder and rectum. Lymphatic spread from tumours in the upper vagina is to the iliac and obturator nodes, whereas that from neoplasms in the lower vagina is to the femoral and inguinal nodes. The current overall 5-year survival rate is about 30%.

The aetiology of vaginal squamous carcinoma is unknown but it has been suggested that long-standing procidentia or the prolonged wearing of a pessary may be of some aetiological importance. This may well be true but these factors are of little importance in current practice. The role of HPV infection in the aetiology of vaginal carcinoma is currently undetermined.

CLEAR-CELL ADENOCARCINOMA

Vaginal neoplasms of this type used to be of extreme rarity but their incidence increased in the cohort of girls and young women who had been exposed prenatally to DES. Approximately one in 1500 women exposed to DES during the first 18 weeks of their prenatal life will develop a clear-cell adenocarcinoma, the tumour usually becoming apparent between the ages of 14 and 23 years, most commonly in girls aged 17–19 years. The tumour almost certainly originates in pre-existing vaginal adenosis and is therefore of müllerian origin. In women who have not been exposed to DES, the tumours usually develop between the ages of 40 and 50 years.

A clear-cell adenocarcinoma usually develops in the upper third of the vagina and may form a polypoid, nodular or papillary mass. Histologically (Figure 2.3), there is a complex mixture of solid papillary, tubular and cystic patterns, the solid areas being formed by sheets of cells with clear cytoplasm and the tubules being lined by 'hobnail' cells which have large nuclei that protrude into the tubular lumen.

The tumour spreads by local invasion, through the lymphatics and through the bloodstream. Although the pelvic nodes are commonly the site of metastases, there is a surprisingly high incidence of spread to the supraclavicular nodes. Blood-borne dissemination is principally to the lungs. Treatment is by radical surgery and the overall 5-year survival rate is 80%.

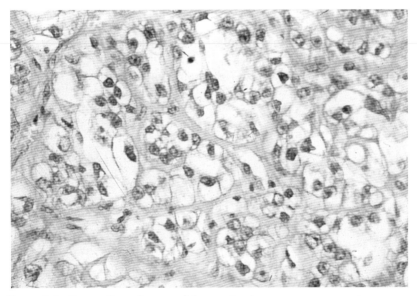

Figure 2.3. Clear-cell carcinoma of the vagina in a woman exposed prenatally to diethylstilbestrol: the neoplasm is composed of small acini lined by clear cells or 'hobnail' cells set in a fibrous stroma (reproduced with permission from Fox and Buckley, *Atlas of Gynaecological Pathology*, published by MTP Press)

OTHER ADENOCARCINOMAS AND RARE NEOPLASMS

Other primary adenocarcinomas of the vagina may be of intestinal type, endometrioid type, developing in vaginal endometriosis or of endocervical pattern developing in vaginal adenosis (Figure 2.4). Rare cases of primary serous carcinoma of the vagina and carcinoma of Gartner's duct have been reported. Non-neoplastic conditions, such as a prolapsed fallopian tube (Figure 2.5) and non-specific granulation tissue (Figure 2.6), may clinically mimic a malignancy.

Primary malignant melanoma of the vagina is rare, metastatic malignant melanoma being more common. The prognosis of primary malignant melanoma is poor. The mean survival rate is only 15 months, being worst in tumours with a high mitotic count.

SARCOMA BOTRYOIDES

The term 'sarcoma botryoides' is applied to the rare embryonal rhabdomyosarcoma of the vagina, a tumour which most commonly occurs in the first 5 years of life. The neoplasm arises from the connective tissues of the vaginal wall and tends to form a polypoid mass of greyish-red haemorrhagic tissue which may fill and protrude from the vagina. Histologically, there is typically a widely dispersed population of pleomorphic immature mesenchymal cells, rhabdomyoblasts and striated muscle cells set in an abundant oedematous or myxoid stroma (Figure 2.7). The epithelium covering the tumour is bland and the neoplastic cells tend to be condensed below this to form a 'cambium' layer. Vaginal sarcoma botryoides infiltrates locally into the pelvic tissues and has a poor prognosis.

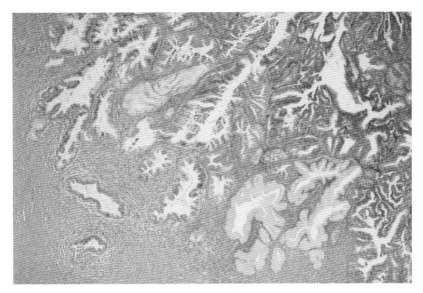

Figure 2.4. Primary mucus-secreting, focally intestinal-type adenocarcinoma of the vagina developing in a case of vaginal adenosis

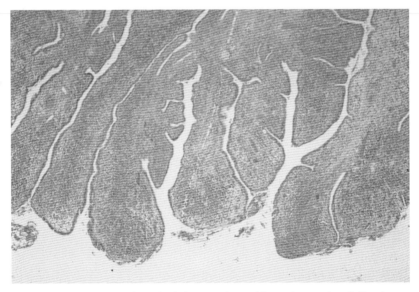

Figure 2.5. Fallopian tube which has prolapsed into the vagina following hysterectomy; the fimbria are swollen and chronically inflamed

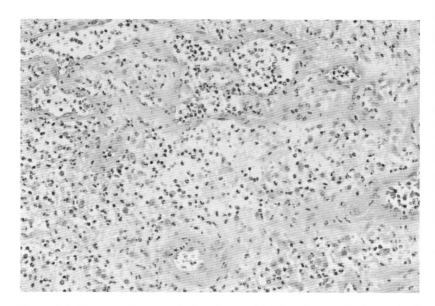

Figure 2.6. Non-specific granulation tissue which has formed in the vaginal vault following hysterectomy; the lesion formed cushions of friable, haemorrhagic tissue, which was mistaken for recurrent carcinoma

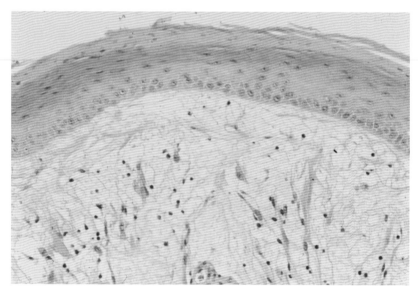

Figure 2.7. Sarcoma botryoides or embryonal rhabdomyosarcoma: the covering squamous epithelium is of normal appearance; strap-like striated muscle cells are present in the underlying soft tissue

3 The cervix

Physiological changes in the cervix

ECTOPY OR ECTROPION

In the prepubertal girl, the squamocolumnar junction lies around the external os or on the ectocervix. At the time of puberty, in pregnancy (particularly the first pregnancy) and in many steroid contraceptive users, changes in the hormonal milieu result in an alteration in the shape and an increase in the bulk of the cervix. These changes result in eversion of the endocervical epithelium with the squamocolumnar junction being carried passively further out on to the anatomical ectocervix. This rim of endocervical tissue forms an ectopy or ectropion exposed around the external os. The ectopy appears red through the thin covering epithelium and the surface is villous (Figure 3.1).

The exposure of the delicate endocervical epithelium to the acid environment of the vagina leads to squamous metaplasia with the squamous epithelial cells differentiating from pluripotential uncommitted cells, through an intermediate stage referred to as reserve cell hyperplasia. Squamous metaplasia is a protective mechanism in which relatively fragile endocervical columnar epithelium is replaced by a more robust squamous epithelium.

The metaplastic squamous epithelium may occlude the mouths of the endocervical crypts with the resultant formation of retention cysts or Nabothian follicles (Figure 3.2). This process also restores the position of the squamocolumnar junction to the external os. The area of squamous metaplasia is termed the transformation zone. This is the site at which the majority of cervical neoplasms arise. In young women, the transformation zone lies where it develops, on the ectocervix, but after the age of 30 years there is an increasing tendency, because of shrinkage of the soft tissue of the cervix, for the squamocolumnar junction to be retracted and come to lie within the endocervical canal; hence, that area of epithelium which formed the transformation zone is also withdrawn to within the canal. An endocervical squamocolumnar junction is a virtually constant finding after the menopause.

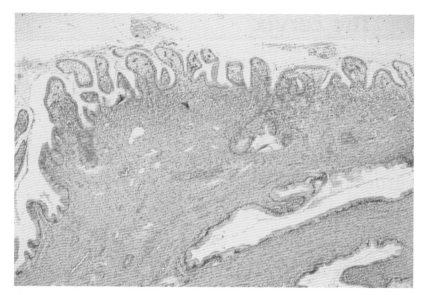

Figure 3.1. A cervical ectopy showing the villous surface

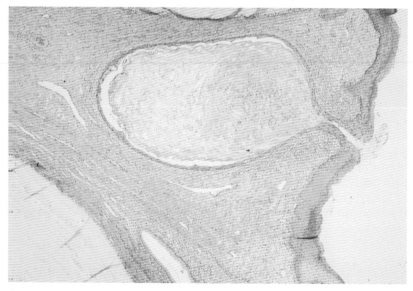

Figure 3.2. A mature transformation zone in which squamous metaplasia of the surface epithelium has obstructed some of the endocervical crypts to create obstructive cysts (Nabothian follicles)

PREGNANCY

In pregnancy, in addition to the development of an ectopy, there is a spongy enlargement of the cervix because of congestion and oedema. Surface maturation of the squamous epithelium is absent because of progesterone predominance in the hormonal milieu. Focal decidualisation of the stroma is common (Figure 3.3) and may be detected at colposcopy. Less commonly, Arias Stella change (see page 66)occurs in the epithelium of the endocervical crypts (Figure 3.4). The columnar epithelium of the ectopy or endocervical canal often undergoes a form of hyperplasia characterised by tightly packed glands or tubules lined by flattened or cuboidal cells. This condition of microglandular hyperplasia (Figure 3.5) is, in most cases, only a microscopic change, although it may on rare occasions form polypoid nodules which bleed on touch. Similar changes may occur in hormonal contraceptive users and with progestogen therapy.

Inflammatory disease of the cervix

Cervical inflammation (cervicitis) may occur as an isolated lesion or as part of a more widespread inflammatory process in the genital tract. The histological appearances are, however, remarkably stereotyped and often give no clue as to the aetiology (Figure 3.6). Inflammation may be acute, active chronic or chronic and chronic inflammation may be granulomatous or (much more commonly) non-granulomatous. There is a normal population of plasma cells and lymphocytes in the stroma adjacent to the external cervical os and these often lead to an unwarranted diagnosis of cervicitis. Hence, the recognition of an inflammatory process depends upon the presence not only of inflammatory cells but also on the finding of associated changes, such as a reduction in mucus secretion, infiltration of the epithelium by inflammatory cells, ulceration, the formation of granulation tissue, fibrosis, the development of lymphoid follicles with germinal centres or granuloma formation.

Acute inflammation is characterised by oedema and congestion, the presence in the stroma and crypts of polymorphonuclear leucocytes and an acute inflammatory exudate. In severe cases, there may be abscess formation and ulceration of the surface epithelium. In persistent or active chronic inflammation the infiltrate becomes plasma-lymphocytic and histiocytic with scanty polymorphonuclear leucocytes, while in some chronic infections lymphoid follicles or granulomas are a characteristic feature.

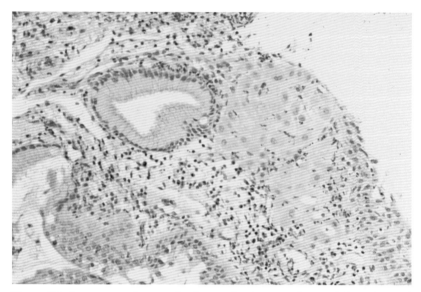

Figure 3.3. Pregnancy changes in the cervix: the cytoplasm of the enlarged stromal cells, to the right, is eosinophilic; this is decidual change

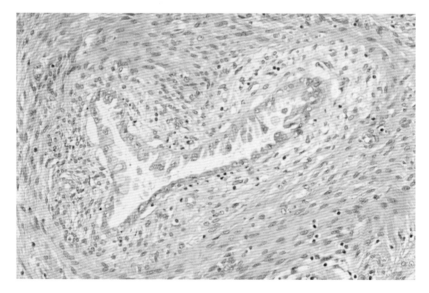

Figure 3.4. Pregnancy changes in the cervix: the crypt is lined by a columnar epithelium in which there is nuclear enlargement and pleomorphism; this is Arias Stella change similar to that which occurs in the endometrium

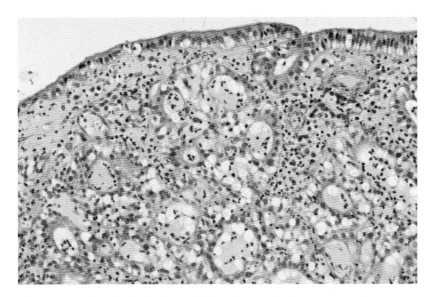

Figure 3.5. Microglandular hyperplasia: the cervical stroma contains a cluster of small, closely packed glands lined by epithelium of endocervical type; polymorphonuclear leucocytes are present in the stroma

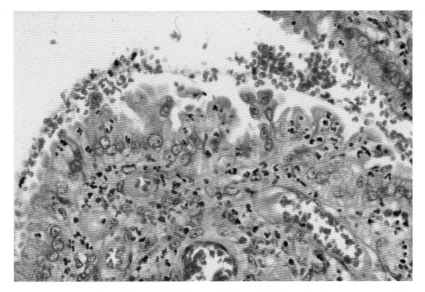

Figure 3.6. Reactive changes in the cervical epithelium in the presence of active inflammation; the epithelial cells are enlarged, there is mild nuclear pleomorphism and some cellular stratification

NON-INFECTIVE INFLAMMATION

Inflammation occurs following surgery, parturition, cryosurgery, laser therapy, cautery, the use of douches or ointments and in association with the presence of an intrauterine contraceptive device. The cervix often becomes inflamed if there is a prolapse and this is particularly marked if ulceration occurs. This inflammation is due to a combination of tissue ischaemia following alterations in the blood supply to the cervix as it descends and rubbing from clothing and is termed decubital ulceration.

INFECTIVE INFLAMMATION

Many infections of the cervix are of a non-specific polymicrobial nature. Bacterial infections tend particularly to involve the endocervix or an ectopy, partly because the columnar epithelium in these sites offers less resistance to infection than does the stratified squamous epithelium of the ectocervix and partly because organisms sequestrated in the cervical crypts may not be affected by either systemic or local therapeutic agents. Chronic cervical inflammation occurs, particularly when there is obstruction to and stasis of cervical secretions and is therefore encountered when the vagina is obstructed by a foreign body or tumour or when the endocervical canal is blocked by a neoplasm, polyp or stricture. The resultant scarring and fibrosis leads to further crypt destruction, thus increasing the obstruction and perpetuating the inflammatory process. The organisms most commonly isolated in such circumstances include coliforms, commensals, mycoplasma, *Gardnerella vaginalis* and *Chlamydia* but their role in initiating the inflammation is uncertain.

VIRAL INFECTIONS

Herpes simplex virus type 2

Herpetic infection of the cervix is most common in teenagers and young adults and is usually associated with infection of the vulva and vagina. Symptoms develop 3–7 days after inoculation and are most severe in primary infections. Although healing is usually rapid and complete, recurrences are frequent and an asymptomatic infected state may develop.

Focal necrosis of the squamous epithelium of the cervix leads to the development of shallow ulcers and, rarely, to the development of a necrotising cervicitis or a chronic inflammatory mass, which may be mistaken for a carcinoma.

Human papillomavirus

Cervical infection by HPV, a sexually-transmitted organism, is increasingly common. HPV infection can result in condylomata or flat 'warty' lesions and is of aetiological importance in cervical neoplasia (see pages 43–51).

BACTERIAL INFECTION

Neisseria gonorrhoeae

The squamous epithelium of the ectocervix is relatively resistant to infection by this highly contagious organism. Gonococci can, however, pass through the columnar epithelium of the endocervix to elicit an acute exudative endocervicitis characterised by stromal congestion and oedema and a seropurulent exudate, while the columnar epithelium becomes focally degenerate and ulcerated.

Infection may clear, may become chronic or spread to the endometrium and fallopian tubes. A proportion of women become asymptomatic carriers, while others develop chronic gonococcal cervicitis with pericryptal fibrosis, crypt distortion and stasis of cervical secretions.

Chlamydial infection

Chlamydial infection of the cervix is characterised by the development of a follicular cervicitis (Figure 3.7). The inflammatory infiltrate, which is often heavy, is composed of plasma cells and lymphocytes which form lymphoid follicles with germinal centres. Intraepithelial abscesses and ulceration of the overlying epithelium may develop in severe cases.

Spirochaetal infection

The primary lesion of syphilis occurs in the cervix in up to 40% of cases, where it may form a typical hard, ulcerated chancre but may be asymptomatic. Occasionally, multiple small ulcers form which resemble those seen in herpetic cervicitis and, rarely, a fungating mass resembling a neoplasm may develop. When the chancre lies in the endocervix, the entire cervix may become indurated and oedematous.

The characteristic histological findings are a dense, subepithelial plasma cell infiltrate, a perivascular infiltrate of lymphocytes with endothelial hyperplasia and, in long-standing cases, endarteritis. The mucous patches, but not the condylomata lata of the secondary stage of syphilis, may occur on the cervix but this is an exceptionally rare site for a gumma.

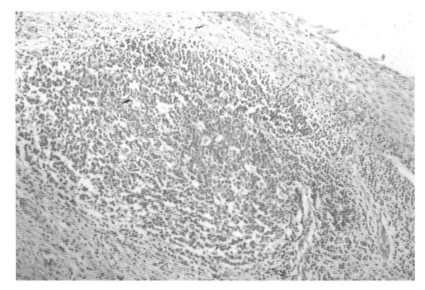

Figure 3.7. Follicular cervicitis: in addition to a diffuse chronic inflammatory cell infiltrate, there is a lymphoid follicle with a germinal centre; the appearances are highly suggestive of chlamydial infection (reproduced with permission from Fox and Buckley, *Atlas of Gynaecological Pathology*, published by MTP Press)

PROTOZOAL AND OTHER INFECTIONS

Trichomonas vaginalis

Infection of the vagina and cervix by *T. vaginalis* are inseparable. The mucosa of the infected cervix is reddened and the underlying vessels are ectatic, appearing as red spots and leading to the descriptive term, a 'strawberry' cervix. The epithelium is infiltrated by polymorphonuclear leucocytes and is partly desquamated with the underlying stroma containing chronic inflammatory cells (Figure 3.8). In many cases, the infection resolves following treatment but in others it may become chronic as the endocervical crypts act as a reservoir of infection.

Schistosomiasis

Schistosomiasis of the cervix is rarely seen in the UK but it is a common genital tract pathogen in some areas of the world. Cervical infection leads to the development of a bulky indurated cervix or a polypoidal mass and there is a granulomatous response to the ova. Progressive fibrosis may cause gross cervical distortion.

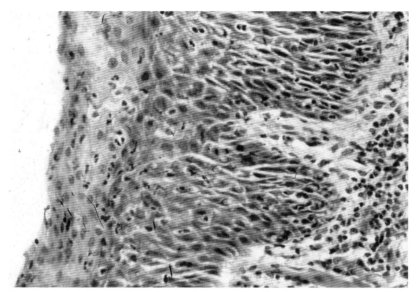
Figure 3.8. Trichomonal cervicitis: the superficial layers of the squamous epithelium of the ectocervix are infiltrated by neutrophil polymorphonucleocytes and there is cellular damage; the underlying stroma is infiltrated by lymphocytes and plasma cells (reproduced with permission from Fox and Buckley, *Atlas of Gynaecological Pathology*, published by MTP Press)

Cervical polyps

Cervical polyps are common and arise in 95% of cases from the endocervix. An endocervical polyp represents a focal overgrowth of hyperplastic endocervical epithelium and its underlying stroma but the cause of this overgrowth is unknown. The polyps form pedunculated, round or ovoid masses of pinkish tissue which grow into the endocervical canal. Histologically, they have a surface epithelium of columnar endocervical-type epithelium which forms crypt-like infoldings into the stroma of the polyp (Figure 3.9). Squamous metaplasia of the surface epithelium is common. Endocervical polyps occur most frequently in women aged 30–50 years and there is no risk of malignant change.

Condylomata of the cervix

Cervical warts or condyloma acuminata have long been recognised but it is only more recently that the flat condyloma (also known as 'warty

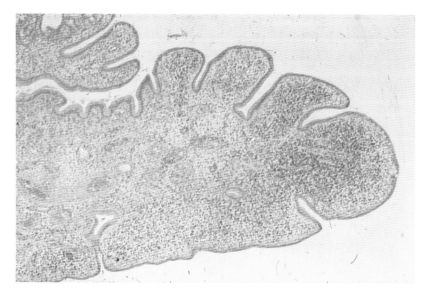

Figure 3.9. A cervical polyp: the polyp is composed of endocervical tissue infiltrated by lymphocytes and containing dilated blood vessels

atypia', 'condyloma planum', 'subclinical' and 'non-condylomatous cervical wart virus infection') has been identified. Both lesions are caused by a sexually transmitted infection with HPV and it is now realised that flat condylomata account for over 90% of HPV infections of the cervix.

Condylomata acuminata are seen as fleshy, pointed papules which are often multiple and sometimes confluent. A flat condyloma (Figure 3.10) is, by contrast, not visible to the naked eye and, although often suggested by an abnormal cervical smear, is detectable only on colposcopy and histology. The hallmark of an HPV infection is the presence, within squamous epithelium, of koilocytes. These cells have enlarged, irregular, hyperchromatic nuclei with a prominent clear perinuclear space (halo) and margination of the cytoplasm (Figure 3.11). Multinucleation and premature individual cell keratinisation (dyskeratosis) are other typical features of HPV infection.

Condylomata occur most commonly in the squamous epithelium of the transformation zone of young women and HPV types 6, 11, 16 or 18 have been identified in a very high proportion of these lesions. Condylomata due to infection with HPV types 6, 11, 42, 43 and 44 almost invariably pursue a benign course. Some regress spontaneously while the remainder may persist, in the absence of treatment, in an

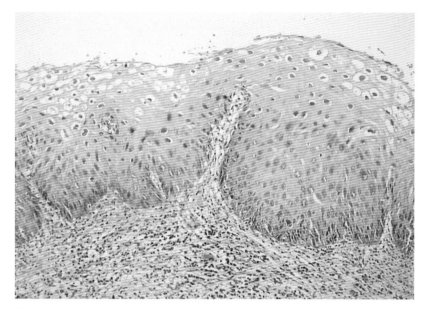

Figure 3.10. Subclinical or non-condylomatous wart virus infection (flat condyloma): the cells in the upper layers of the squamous epithelium are vacuolated and the nuclei are enlarged (koilocytes); there is some basal cell hyperplasia in the deep layers of the epithelium but no nuclear atypia

unchanged state for many years. Condylomata due to HPV strains 16 and 18 are, however, frequently complicated by a superimposed CIN and it should be noted that condylomata due to these strains of HPV are always of the flat variety.

Cervical neoplasms

Squamous carcinomas, adenocarcinomas and adenosquamous carcinomas all occur in the cervix but squamous tumours predominate, to the extent that there is a tendency to think of cervical cancer only in terms of squamous carcinoma. This undoubtedly blurs our understanding of the aetiology, pathogenesis and development of the different tumours.

With the exception of leiomyomas, benign tumours of the cervix are rare but may, clinically, mimic carcinoma. Benign tumours include blue naevus, neurofibroma, ganglioneuroma, haemangioma, lymphangioma, lipoma, rhabdomyoma, mature cystic teratoma, papillary adenofibroma, lipoleiomyoma and endocervical adenomyoma.

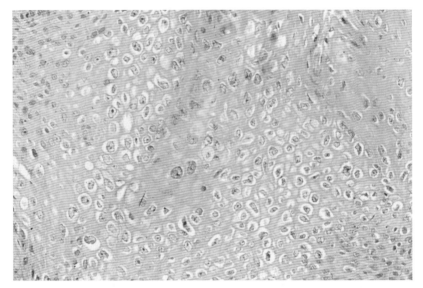

Figure 3.11. Koilocytes: the squamous nuclei are enlarged, pleomorphic and in places 'boat shaped'; the perinuclear cytoplasm is vacuolated

SQUAMOUS NEOPLASIA

Both preinvasive and invasive squamous neoplasms occur. The condition of CIN is thought to represent an intraepithelial neoplasm. This lesion occurs, in the vast majority of cases, in that area of metaplastic squamous epithelium within the transformation zone. CIN may, therefore, develop on the anatomical ectocervix or within the endocervical canal and is a recognised precursor of invasive squamous carcinoma.

Invasive and intraepithelial squamous neoplasia of the cervix have, as might be expected, aetiological factors in common and it is therefore convenient to discuss the aetiology of both conditions together. Some adenocarcinomas and adenosquamous carcinomas appear to share common aetiological factors with squamous carcinomas but other adenocarcinomas have different aetiological correlates.

During the process of metaplasia, the immature squamous epithelium of the transformation zone appears to be particularly susceptible to oncogenic stimuli. Various factors have been identified which may be of aetiological importance in the development of preinvasive and invasive neoplasia of the cervix, although final proof of their significance is still lacking. They can be divided into epidemiological factors and causative agents.

It is almost unknown for CIN or invasive squamous carcinoma of the cervix to develop in women who have never had coitus and the greater the number of sexual partners she or her consort have had and the younger her age at first coitus, the greater her risk of developing cervical carcinoma. There is a relatively high frequency of sexually transmitted disease in women with cervical neoplasia but this may simply be related to the likelihood of a greater number of sexual partners. There is a slightly increased risk of cervical neoplasia in women who use oral contraception and a decreased risk for those using a barrier form of contraception. The protection offered by barrier methods may reflect the fact that exposure of the cervix to seminal plasma results in local immunosuppression but may also indicate the ability of barrier contraception to prevent the transmission of an aetiological agent. Oral contraception allows the transmission of such an agent and also alters the hormonal milieu of the cervix.

Cigarette smoking is an independent risk factor for cervical neoplasia. This may be due to the excretion in the cervical mucus of chemicals derived from tobacco smoke, which are not only capable of exerting a carcinogenic effect but also appear to cause local immunosuppression.

Women infected by the human immunodeficiency virus (HIV) are at particular risk of developing CIN and cervical carcinoma if they are also infected by HPV.

All the epidemiological data indicate that a sexually transmitted agent is implicated in the aetiology of cervical neoplasia and there is now overwhelming evidence that a central role is played by certain types of HPV, particularly types 16 and 18. Infection with these viruses is common in young women but the vast majority of such infections are transient, with the virus being rapidly cleared from the cervix. The women at risk for cervical neoplasia are those in whom the viral infection persists. The reasons for viral persistence in a small proportion of women are unknown but co-factors such as smoking, local immunosuppression and other synergistic viral infections may be of importance.

It is probable that HPV is present in all cervical squamous cell carcinomas and is often integrated into the host genome. Some indication of how these viruses act as oncogenic agents has come from the demonstration that the proteins coded for by the E6 and E7 genes of HPV-16 or -18 combine with and result in the degradation of the tumour-suppressor p53.

CIN usually occurs at a younger age than does squamous carcinoma, which has its peak incidence in women over the age of 45 years. In recent years, although the incidence of carcinoma in women between the ages of 35 and 45 years has declined, the incidence in women under the age of 35 years has increased and there has been little change in the incidence in women over the age of 45 years. There are now less than 1500 deaths a year from cervical cancer in England and Wales, while the incidence of CIN has shown a dramatic increase; this disparity reflects the success of the cervical screening programme.

CERVICAL INTRAEPITHELIAL NEOPLASIA

CIN is a single continuous disease process that is characterised histologically by a failure of the normal process of maturation in the squamous epithelium of the transformation zone, together with a variable degree of nuclear enlargement and pleomorphism. In the UK, CIN is graded into CIN 1 (Figure 3.12), CIN 2 (Figure 3.13) and CIN 3 (Figure 13.14) (Table 3.1) and this terminology is preferred to that of the Bethesda system, which includes flat condylomata within its grading system and simply recognises two entities of 'high- and low-grade squamous intraepithelial lesions' (Table 3.2). In practical terms,

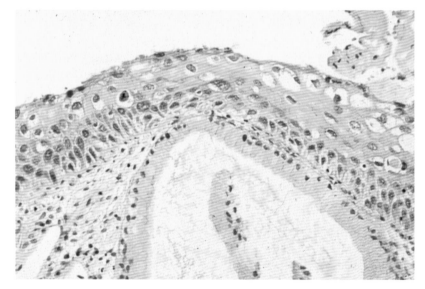

Figure 3.12. Cervical intraepithelial neoplasia (CIN) grades 1 and 2: the nuclei in all layers are enlarged, pleomorphic and hyperchromatic; cytoplasmic maturation is present in the upper two-thirds of the epithelium to the right (CIN 1) but only in the outer-third of the epithelium to the left (CIN 2); note the koilocytes

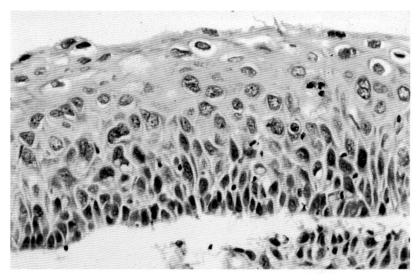

Figure 3.13. Cervical intraepithelial neoplasia grade 2: there is nuclear enlargement, pleomorphism and hyperchromasia at all levels in the epithelium but there is cytoplasmic maturation in the upper half of the epithelium; the koilocytes and multinucleated cells are indicative of human papillomavirus infection

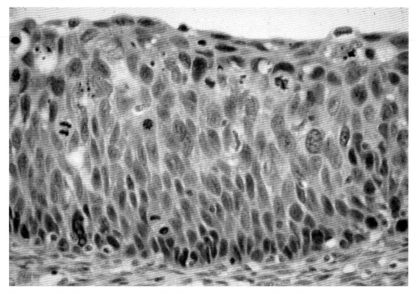

Figure 3.14. Cervical intraepithelial neoplasia grade 3: the nuclei throughout the full thickness of this epithelium are enlarged, pleomorphic and hyperchromatic; there is little or no cytoplasmic maturation (reproduced with permission from *Diagnostic Histopathology of Tumours*, edited by CDM Fletcher, published by Churchill Livingstone)

however, CIN 1 is treated as a low-grade, perhaps spontaneously regressing lesion, while CIN 2 and 3 are conditions warranting more active treatment. This system reflects the likelihood of progression of the disease to invasive carcinoma.

Table 3.1 Grading of cervical intraepithelial neoplasia	
Grade	**Definition**
1	Recognised by mild nuclear abnormalities at all levels of the squamous epithelium but a lack of cytoplasmic maturation of the cells in the lower third of the squamous epithelium
2	Failure of cytoplasmic maturation in the cells in the lower one- to two-thirds of the epithelium and a greater degree of nuclear atypia which persists to the surface of the epithelium
3	Failure of cytoplasmic maturation extends into the upper third of the epithelium or occupies its full thickness and nuclear atypia, of a more severe type, is present throughout the epithelium

Table 3.2 A comparison of the different systems for classifying squamous neoplasia

Term	HPV risk category	Comparison of classification systems		
		2-tiered CIN	Dysplasia/CIS	SIL
Exophytic condyloma	Low risk	–	–	Low grade
Squamous papilloma	Low risk	–	–	Low grade
Flat condyloma	Low & high risk	–	–	Low grade
CIN 1	Low & high risk	Low-grade CIN	Mild dysplasia	Low grade
CIN 2	High risk	High-grade CIN	Moderate dysplasia	High grade
CIN 3	High risk	High-grade CIN	Severe dysplasia/CIS	High grade

CIN = cervical intraepithelial neoplasia; CIS = carcinoma in situ; HPV = human papillomavirus; SIL = squamous intraepithelial lesions

Features indicative of HPV infection are present in many cases, these being the presence of koilocytes, epithelial multinucleation and individual cell keratinisation. These abnormalities are most evident in CIN 1 and 2 and are least apparent in CIN 3 when the virus is incorporated into the cellular genome. CIN 3 is usually assumed to be a squamous intraepithelial neoplasm but can be closely mimicked by a very poorly differentiated adenocarcinoma in situ, which can be recognised only by the use of a mucin stain.

The grade of CIN is rarely uniform throughout the affected area of the transformation zone. Generally, it is of lower grade at the outer ectocervical margin, adjacent to the ectocervical squamous epithelium and of higher grade centrally.

In the transformation zone, metaplasia is not always limited to the surface epithelium and, similarly, CIN may also extend into the underlying endocervical crypts.

When invasion occurs from CIN, it may occur from the surface epithelium or from crypts and, although the epithelium from which invasion has occurred most commonly has the features of CIN 3, invasion may less commonly occur from CIN 1 or 2.

CIN is a precursor of invasive squamous cell carcinoma but not all, or even most, cases of CIN will progress to an invasive neoplasm. It is probable that approximately 35–40% of cases of CIN 3 will evolve into an invasive squamous cell carcinoma within 20 years of diagnosis if untreated. The long-term risk of invasive neoplasia in cases of CIN 1 and 2 is less well defined but in any individual woman with persistent CIN 1 or 2 there is a risk of eventual squamous cell carcinoma.

MICROINVASIVE CARCINOMA (STAGE IA INVASIVE CARCINOMA)

Invasion from squamous or columnar cell intraepithelial neoplasia is first recognised by an increase in the amount of cytoplasm and eosinophilia of the cytoplasm in one or more cells in the basal layer of the epithelium covering the surface of the cervix or lining one or more of the crypts. Subsequently, the deep margin of the epithelium becomes irregular and jagged as tongues of infiltrating cells penetrate the underlying stroma (Figures 3.15 and 3.16), where they evoke a lymphocytic infiltrate and, sometimes, local stromal oedema or fibrosis (desmoplasia).

Although the term 'microinvasive carcinoma' is not included in the FIGO staging definitions for cervical neoplasms, the term is commonly used to describe a degree of invasion that is associated with minimal risk of nodal metastasis and is sufficiently small to treat in many cases by local or conservative means. Microinvasive carcinoma encompasses a small measurable tumour (as described below) and non-confluent tongues or individual cells infiltrating the stroma (early stromal invasion). It may be multifocal or limited to a single focus. It must not exceed 7 mm in its greatest horizontal axis and must not penetrate the stroma for more than 5 mm from the base of the epithelium from which it arises. Stage IA is subdivided into stage IA1, lesions no more than 7 mm in their greatest horizontal axis and no more than 3 mm in

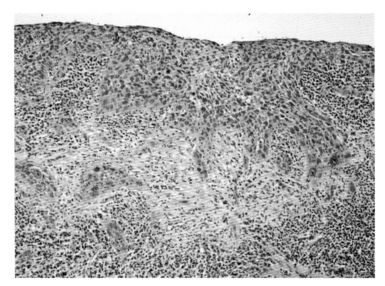

Figure 3.15. 'Early stromal invasion': multiple tongues of eosinophilic staining cells penetrate the cervical stroma from the deep surface of an epithelium in which there are features of cervical intraepithelial neoplasia; note the mild stromal oedema and the lymphocytic response to the invading cells

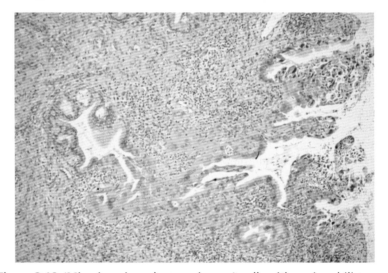

Figure 3.16. 'Microinvasive adenocarcinoma': cells with eosinophilic cytoplasm infiltrate the stroma below and are in continuity with the abnormal mucus-secreting columnar epithelium of endocervical type which lines the crypt, to the right, and covers the surface of the cervix; there is mild oedema and a lymphocytic infiltrate in the surrounding stroma

depth, and stage IA2, lesions no more than 7 mm in their greatest horizontal axis and 3–5 mm in depth. Some restrict use of the term 'microinvasive' to stage IA1 only. With the smallest lesions, a minor degree of lymphatic permeation in the immediate vicinity of the neoplasm does not exclude the lesion from this category. Earlier descriptions of microinvasive carcinoma, in terms only of its depth of penetration, are now regarded as having little value and can be misleading and potentially dangerous. It is also recognised that all carcinomas which are clinically apparent, no matter how small or superficial, should not be regarded as microinvasive.

INVASIVE SQUAMOUS CELL CARCINOMA

Squamous carcinomas constitute about 70% of all malignant cervical neoplasms. They can occur at any age from 17 to 70 years but develop most commonly in women in their sixth or seventh decade.

Squamous carcinoma may develop either on the ectocervix, where it tends to grow in a predominantly exophytic manner to form a papillary or polypoidal mass, or in the endocervical canal, where it commonly expands the cervix to form a hard barrel-shaped mass. Ulceration and necrosis are common features and the tumours often bleed on touch.

Histologically, squamous cell carcinoma infiltrates cervical stroma as a network of anastomosing bands which appear in cross-section as irregular islands with spiky or angular margins. The tumours may be well differentiated (the large-cell keratinising type; Figure 3.17), moderately differentiated (large-cell focally keratinising type) or poorly differentiated (large- or small-cell non-keratinising types; Figure 3.18). As 80% are either moderately or poorly differentiated tumours, well-differentiated neoplasms are the exception rather than the rule.

Squamous cell carcinomas spread locally to invade the uterine body, vagina, bladder and rectum with spread occurring along the paracervical ligaments to the lateral side walls of the pelvis, surrounding and compressing the ureters as they traverse the paracervical region. Lymphatic spread is to the paracervical, iliac, obturator and para-aortic nodes but dissemination by this route does not occur methodically and an absence of metastases in the iliac nodes is no guarantee that tumour will not be present in para-aortic nodes. Blood-borne spread is a late phenomenon and is principally to the liver, lungs and skeleton.

Delineation of prognostic factors for women with invasive cervical squamous carcinoma is probably only of real value in those with stage Ib or IIa disease. In such cases, the two most important factors governing the prognosis are the extent of the local disease and the presence or otherwise of nodal metastases. The extent of the local

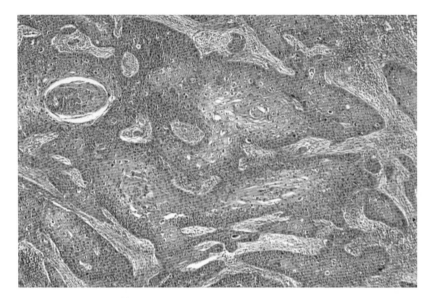

Figure 3.17. Well-differentiated, keratinising squamous cell carcinoma; note the jagged infiltrating margin to the right

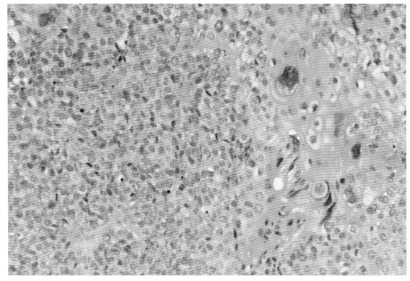

Figure 3.18. Focally keratinising, poorly differentiated squamous cell carcinoma

disease is usually defined by clinical examination, including scans (Table 3.3) but, to a very significant extent, the prognosis depends upon whether nodal metastases are present or not. Tumour differentiation is probably not of prognostic significance while factors such as tumour size and vascular space invasion are surrogates for the risk of nodal metastasis rather than independent prognostic indices.

Table 3.3 FIGO staging of carcinoma of the cervix	
Stage	Definition
0	Preinvasive carcinoma (CIN 3, CGIN 3, carcinoma in situ)
I	Carcinoma confined to the cervix (extension to the corpus should be disregarded for staging purposes)
Ia	Measured stromal invasion with a maximum depth of 5 mm and no more than 7 mm in its greatest width
Ia1	Measured stromal invasion up to 3 mm in depth and no more than 7 mm in its greatest width
Ia2	Measured stromal invasion 3–5 mm in depth and no more than 7 mm in width
Ib	Clinically apparent lesions confined to the cervix or preclinical lesions greater than stage Ia
Ib1	Lesions no greater than 4 cm in size
Ib2	Lesions greater than 4 cm in size
II	Invasive carcinoma that extends beyond the cervix but has not reached either the lateral pelvic wall: involvement of the vagina is limited to the upper two-thirds
IIa	No obvious parametrial involvement
IIb	Obvious parametrial involvement
III	Invasive carcinoma that extends to either lateral pelvic wall and/or the lower-third of the vagina: includes all cases with a hydronephrosis or non-functioning kidney
IIIa	No extension to the pelvic side wall but lower-third of the vagina involved
IIIb	Extension to the pelvic side wall, hydronephrosis or non-functioning kidney
IV	Carcinoma extends beyond the true pelvis or has involved the mucosa of the urinary bladder or rectum
IVa	Spread of tumour to the adjacent organs
IVb	Spread to distant organs

GLANDULAR NEOPLASIA

Both adenocarcinoma in situ and invasive adenocarcinoma of the cervix are recognised but the relationship between these two conditions is much less clearly defined than is that between CIN and squamous carcinoma of the cervix. Adenocarcinomas currently constitute 12–16% of all cervical neoplasms and this proportion is rising. Whether this reflects a genuine increase in the incidence of these tumours or is due to a reduction in the number of squamous carcinomas is uncertain.

Many adenocarcinomas are found in women with aetiological factors similar to those for squamous carcinoma and HPV strains 16 and 18 have been identified in adenocarcinomas. Long-term use of the oral contraceptive pill has been particularly implicated as a co-factor in cervical adenocarcinoma.

CERVICAL GLANDULAR INTRAEPITHELIAL NEOPLASIA (ADENOCARCINOMA IN SITU)

High-grade cervical glandular intraepithelial neoplasia (CGIN) (severe glandular dysplasia/adenocarcinoma in situ) occurs in the mucus-secreting columnar epithelium on the surface of a cervical ectopy, within the endocervical canal or within endocervical crypts. It is recognised histologically by:

- stratification of the epithelial cells
- loss of nuclear polarity and mucin-secreting capacity
- an increase in nucleocytoplasmic ratios, cellular pleomorphism, nuclear hyperchromatism
- the presence of numerous, sometimes atypical, mitoses (Figure 3.19).

An increasing complexity of the glandular pattern is often, although not invariably, present. The least well-differentiated forms come to resemble squamous CIN 3. Lesser degrees of epithelial abnormality are recognised, to which the term low-grade CGIN (Figure 3.20) is applied, although their assessment is highly subjective.

The relationship between CGIN and invasive adenocarcinoma of the cervix and the risk of progression from one to the other is not established. In certain cases, the origin of an adenocarcinoma from an in situ lesion can be traced but an accompanying adenocarcinoma in situ is not necessarily identified adjacent to all adenocarcinomas. In particular, the clinical significance of low-grade CGIN is uncertain.

ADENOCARCINOMA

There are several histological types of adenocarcinoma, of which by far the most common is the endocervical type, in which the constituent cells bear an anarchic resemblance to those of the normal endocervix.

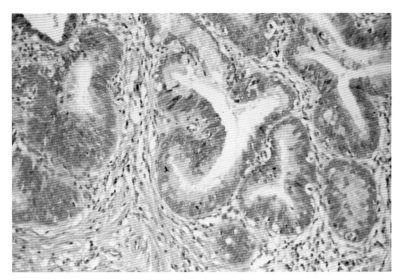

Figure 3.19. Cervical glandular intraepithelial neoplasia grade 3 (adenocarcinoma in situ): the crypts are lined by columnar epithelium which is focally stratified, the nuclei enlarged, hyperchromatic and pleomorphic, and mitoses are present (reproduced with permission from *Diagnostic Histopathology of Tumors*, edited by CDM Fletcher, published by Churchill Livingstone)

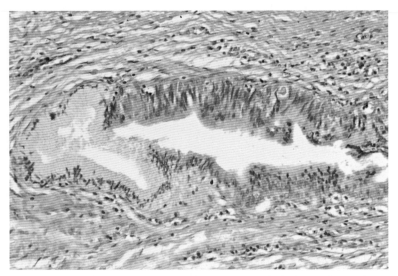

Figure 3.20. Low grade cervical glandular intraepithelial neoplasia: the crypt lining to the left is normal but there is an abrupt transition to a stratified epithelium with a minor degree of nuclear enlargement and hyperchromasia

Endocervical adenocarcinoma

These tumours may be well, moderately or poorly differentiated. The well-differentiated tumours form glandular acini and branching clefts and crypts and the cells resemble those of the endocervix to a greater or lesser extent (Figure 3.21). Loss of differentiation is characterised by the loss of the glandular pattern and mucus-secreting capacity. The least well-differentiated forms assume a solid rather than a glandular pattern and thus come, histologically, to resemble a squamous carcinoma, with which they may be confused.

Some endocervical adenocarcinomas are extremely well differentiated and have a surprisingly bland histological appearance. They are known as 'minimal deviation adenocarcinomas' or 'adenoma malignum' (Figure 3.22).

Clear-cell carcinoma

Cervical neoplasms of this type are identical to the clear-cell adeno-carcinoma of the vagina (Figure 2.3) and, although occurring typically in DES-exposed women, are by no means limited to this group.

Endometrioid adenocarcinoma

This term is used to describe carcinomas which are identical histologically with those adenocarcinomas that develop in the endometrium. In addition to the typical endometrioid adenocarcinomas, minimal deviation endometrioid adenocarcinoma is also described. All forms are uncommon in the cervix.

Rare cervical adenocarcinomas

These include papillary serous adenocarcinoma, which is histologically identical to a papillary serous adenocarcinoma of the ovary; enteric adenocarcinomas, which resemble intestinal adenocarcinomas (Figure 3.23) and are probably derived from foci of gastrointestinal metaplasia and mesonephric adenocarcinomas which arise from remnants of the mesonephric duct. Adenoid cystic carcinoma, which typically develops in postmenopausal women, and adenoid basal carcinoma, which is usually associated with CIN, are also rare malignancies of the cervix.

CARCINOMA OF MIXED PATTERN

About 8–10% of cervical carcinomas show evidence of differentiation along more than one cell line. Most commonly, these are adeno-squamous carcinomas (Figure 3.24) and the diagnosis is made only

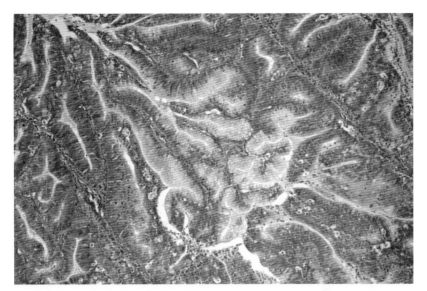

Figure 3.21. Moderately differentiated adenocarcinoma of endocervical type; note the branching clefts or crypts and the reduction in mucus secretion in the peripheral glands

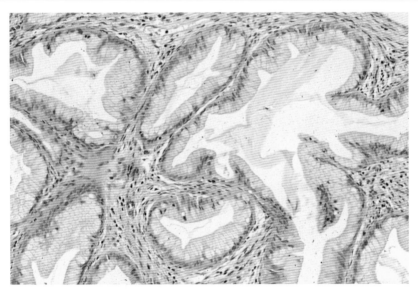

Figure 3.22. Minimal deviation adenocarcinoma of endocervical type: the crypts are of irregular shape but there is minimal cytological atypia

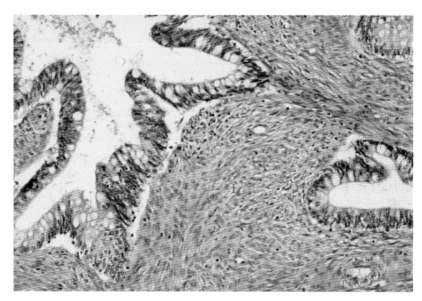

Figure 3.23. Adenocarcinoma of intestinal type: the epithelium is characterised by the presence of goblet cells and mucins of intestinal type

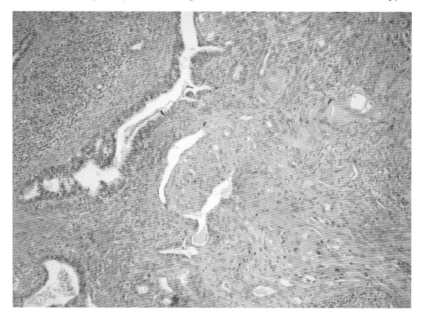

Figure 3.24. Adenosquamous carcinoma: the tumour has two distinct but closely intermingled components; to the left there are well-defined glands, while to the right there is large-cell, focally keratinising squamous differentiation

when histological examination of the tumour is carried out, as they are similar in gross appearance to squamous and adenocarcinomas. These are aggressive neoplasms with a rather poor prognosis.

ENDOCRINE TUMOURS

These neoplasms comprise small-cell carcinomas, large-cell neuro-endocrine tumours and carcinoid tumours. They constitute, in total, about 2% of cases of malignant cervical disease and occur most commonly in the fifth decade of life. They are of neuroendocrine origin and are highly aggressive tumours. They may coexist with adeno-carcinomas (Figure 3.25). The treatment differs from that of most other cervical neoplasms in being primarily chemotherapeutic. Their recognition is, therefore, of particular importance.

MALIGNANT MELANOMA

Malignant melanomas are extremely uncommon but tend to develop in women between the ages of 50 and 70 years. Their prognosis is extremely poor and they must be distinguished from metastatic melanoma, which is more common, and benign pigmented lesions of the cervix.

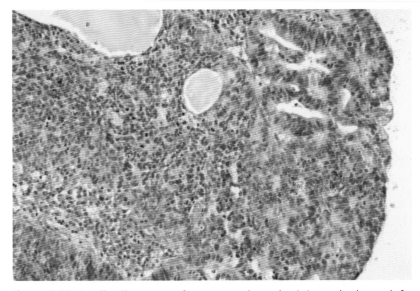

Figure 3.25. Small-cell tumour of neuroectodermal origin to the lower left and adenocarcinoma to the upper right

SARCOMAS

Soft-tissue tumours of the cervix are extremely rare but include stromal sarcomas, resembling low-grade endometrial stromal sarcomas and embryonal rhabdomyosarcomas, the majority of which occur in young women.

METASTATIC CARCINOMAS

Metastatic tumours in the cervix are rare but direct spread from tumours of the vagina, uterine body, bladder, urethra and large bowel are not uncommon. Metastases may come from ovary, colon, stomach, breast, bronchus, kidney, renal pelvis or fallopian tube.

4 The endometrium

Histology of the endometrium

DURING THE MENSTRUAL CYCLE

During the follicular phase of the menstrual cycle (Figure 4.1), when estrogen levels are rising, the various elements of the functional layer of the endometrium proliferate. The glands are at first straight and narrow but become slightly tortuous during the latter part of this phase, when the rate of glandular growth outstrips that of the stroma. The glands are lined by columnar cells with basally situated nuclei and there may be a minor degree of multilayering in the late proliferative phase. The stroma is cellular and, because the stromal cells have little cytoplasm, often presents a 'naked nuclei' appearance. Mitotic figures are present in both glands and stroma throughout the proliferative phase.

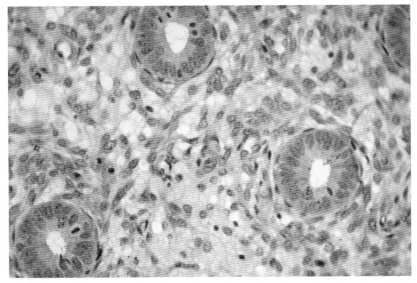

Figure 4.1. Endometrium in the early proliferative phase: the glands, which are straight and narrow, are set in a delicate cellular stroma

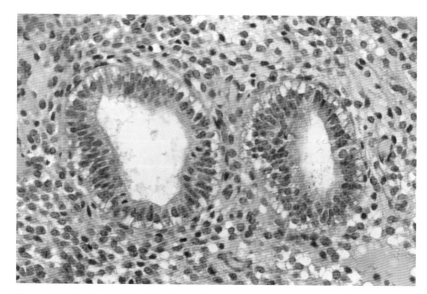

Figure 4.2. Endometrium in the early secretory phase: there are clear subnuclear vacuoles in the glandular epithelial cells (reproduced with permission from Fox and Buckley, *Atlas of Gynaecological Pathology*, published by MTP Press)

In the average cycle, ovulation occurs at about the 14th day with the endometrium then entering, under the influence of rising progesterone levels, the early secretory phase. The morphological changes that characterise the early secretory phase take 24–36 hours to develop. The glands increase slightly in diameter during this period and become somewhat more tortuous. Mitotic figures are still present in the glandular epithelium but decrease progressively in number as progesterone exerts its anti-estrogenic effect. The defining feature of the early secretory phase, clearly apparent 48 hours after ovulation, is the appearance of glycogen-containing subnuclear vacuoles in the glands (Figure 4.2). These vacuoles, when present uniformly in 50% or more of the glands, are taken as being definite evidence that ovulation has occurred. The early secretory phase lasts for about 4 days and between the 5th and 9th postovulatory days the endometrium is in the mid-secretory phase of the cycle (Figure 4.3). The subnuclear vacuoles move to a supranuclear position and secrete their contents into the gland lumina, the nuclei of the glands returning to a basal position. Glandular secretion is at a peak during this period and the glands become increasingly dilated and tortuous.

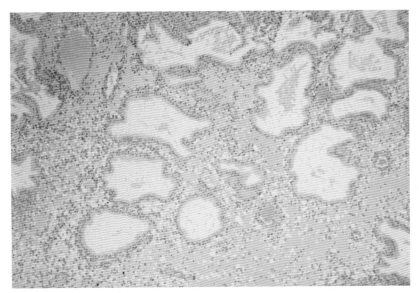

Figure 4.3. Endometrium in the mid-secretory phase: the glands are distended by secretions and are rather angular; the stroma is oedematous

During the mid-secretory phase the stroma is markedly oedematous, largely because of the hormonally-induced increases in both blood flow through and hydrostatic pressure in the endometrial capillary complexes.

At the 10th post-ovulatory day, the endometrium passes into the late secretory phase (Figure 4.4). Glandular secretion diminishes and the glands tend to collapse and become increasingly tortuous. The stromal oedema regresses and the stromal cells take on a predecidual appearance, becoming plump with abundant eosinophilic cytoplasm and small nuclei. The predecidual cells appear first as a mantle around the spiral arteries which, after being previously inconspicuous, are now well developed and prominent. Later, predecidual change is seen in the cells surrounding the glands and in those lying directly below the surface epithelium. Towards the end of the late secretory phase, the stroma consists largely of sheets of predecidual cells which are infiltrated by granulated lymphocytes. The lymphocytes increase in number as the endometrium undergoes menstrual changes, characterised by crumbling, necrosis, infiltration with neutrophil polymorphonuclear leucocytes, glandular collapse and haemorrhage.

It will be appreciated that, throughout the proliferative phase of the cycle, the endometrium shows a rather inconsistent pattern and thus

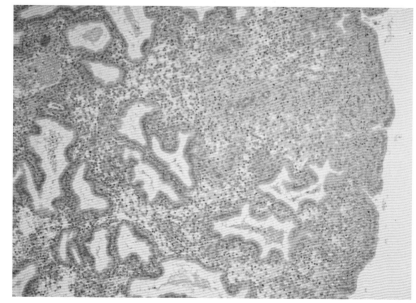

Figure 4.4. Endometrium in the late secretory phase: the glands have a serrated outline, having collapsed after secreting their contents, and the spiral arteries, which are cuffed by decidualised stromal cells, are prominent

an accurate estimation of the day of the menstrual cycle is not possible. After ovulation, the endometrium shows an orderly pattern of time-related changes, which allows for a relatively precise estimate, to within 24–48 hours, of the stage of the cycle.

PREGNANCY

In pregnancy, decidualisation of the stroma persists, the glands become hypersecretory (Figure 4.5) and there is variable vacuolation of the glandular epithelial cells. This may be termed Arias-Stella change (Figure 4.6). The latter change may be seen when the pregnancy is intrauterine and sometimes in ectopic pregnancy

AFTER THE MENOPAUSE

Estrogen levels diminish quite abruptly in many women at the time of the menopause and this results in endometrial atrophy, the endo-metrium becoming shallow, the glands small and inactive and the stroma compact (Figure 4.7). In some women, however, estrogen

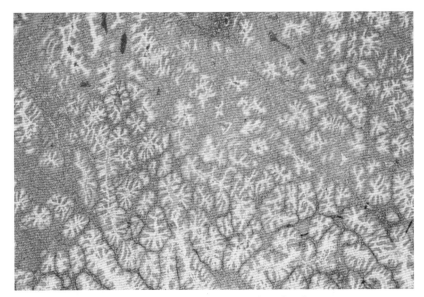

Figure 4.5. Endometrium in early pregnancy: the glands are hypersecretory, enlarged and appear closely packed and stellate

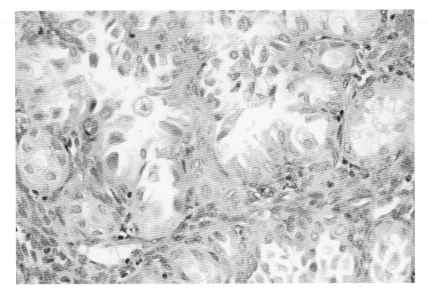

Figure 4.6. Endometrium in pregnancy: the cells lining the glands are hypersecretory, as shown by the presence of cellular enlargement and vacuolation of the cytoplasm

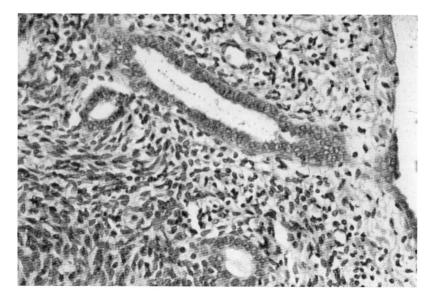

Figure 4.7. Postmenopausal, shallow, inactive endometrium: there is neither proliferative nor secretory activity; the glands are narrow and the stroma is compact (reproduced with permission from Fox and Buckley, *Atlas of Gynaecological Pathology*, published by MTP Press)

levels show a more gradual decline and there may be a rather irregular pattern of proliferation, with mitotic activity still being discernible for up to 2 years after cessation of ovulation. Gradually, however, this low-grade stimulation ceases and the presence of mitotic figures in the endometrium more than 3 years after the menopause is a clear indication of either an abnormal source of endogenous estrogens or the administration of exogenous estrogens.

In a high proportion of postmenopausal women the endometrial glands are, either focally or diffusely, cystically dilated (Figure 4.8), such glands being lined by a single layer of flattened epithelial cells. The incidence of such cystic change increases progressively with advancing age, probably due to blockage of glands during the process of endometrial atrophy and condensation. The cystically dilated glands may, on occasion, become polypoid.

Functional abnormalities of the endometrium

It is usual to distinguish between those abnormalities of endometrial morphology that are secondary to hormonal disturbances and are

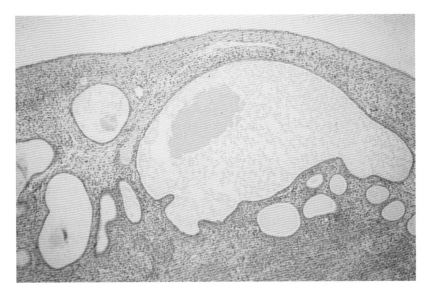

Figure 4.8. Cystic change in an atrophic, postmenopausal endometrium: some of the glands are cystically dilated and are lined by an attenuated epithelium in which there is neither proliferative nor secretory activity

sometimes known as functional disorders of the endometrium, although the term has little to commend it, and those in which there is a primary disease process within the endometrium. Functional abnormalities of the endometrium fall into two main groups: those in which there are inadequacies of hormonal stimulation and those in which such stimulation is excessive.

LOW ESTROGEN STATES

In the absence of ovarian follicular development, there is no estrogen secretion and hence an absence of endometrial growth and proliferation. In such women, the endometrium is shallow and inactive and the uterus is lined only by endometrium of basal type. This is normal after the menopause but is seen in such pathological processes as gonadal dysgenesis, premature menopause, 17-hydroxylase deficiency, gonadotrophin-resistant ovary syndrome and hypogonadotrophic hypogonadism.

HIGH ESTROGEN STATES

The secretory phase of the menstrual cycle is remarkably constant at 14 days and most variation in cycle length is due to changes in the length of the proliferative or follicular phase, which is considered to be abnormally long only when it exceeds 21 days. The endometrium in such cycles may be of normal appearance or may show nothing more than an increased stratification of the glandular epithelium and a mild increase in volume of the endometrium; there are no significant consequences of these minor changes. Menstruation will, however, be less frequent than normal and periods may be irregular.

In some circumstances, ovarian follicular development is not followed by ovulation. As a consequence of continued estrogen secretion by the developing follicle or follicles, the endometrium will continue to grow in an uninterrupted fashion and will eventually become hyperplastic. This condition is discussed in more detail below.

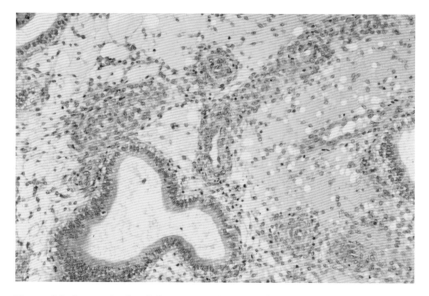

Figure 4.9. Stromal–glandular maturation asynchrony in luteal phase insufficiency: the spiral arteries show early cuffing by decidual stromal cells and are consistent in appearance with the ninth postovulatory day; the glands are consistent with the fourth postovulatory day

LOW PROGESTERONE STATES

Low progesterone states are a natural consequence of failure of normal follicular maturation and of ovulation. In some women, however, less profound deficiencies occur as ovulation is followed by inadequate development of the corpus luteum with resulting progesterone deficiency. These women, described as having 'luteal phase insufficiency' or 'inadequate secretory phase', complain of a variety of symptoms, among which the most common are premenstrual spotting (the loss of small amounts of blood), prolonged menstruation and infertility. Progesterone deficiency may affect the endometrium in one of the following ways:

- a delay in the development of secretory changes following ovulation, so that the endometrium appears to be less mature than suggested by the date of the woman's cycle

- a discrepancy between the maturation of the glands and stroma, with the stroma appearing to be more mature than the glands (dyssynchrony) (Figure 4.9)

- a variable degree of secretory change in different glands in the same tissue, also known as 'irregular ripening' (Figure 4.10).

EXOGENOUS HORMONE EFFECTS

Many of the functional abnormalities of the endometrium may be mimicked by exogenous hormones given to a woman for therapeutic or contraceptive purposes. Thus, the administration of estrogen, unopposed by a progestogen, may result in the development of a simple, complex or atypical endometrial hyperplasia or even a carcinoma (see below).

Progestogens may so inhibit endogenous estrogenic activity that the endometrium can eventually become shallow and atrophic. In women with a progestogen-impregnated intrauterine contraceptive device, the hormone mediated changes may be limited to, or most conspicuous at the device contact site, where there may also be focal inflammation due to mechanical irritation (Figure 4.11).

The changes in the endometrium which accompany the use of a combined steroid contraceptive pill vary greatly according to the dose of hormone administered, the relative potency of the steroids included in the combination or their duration of use. The appearances may mimic those of luteal phase insufficiency or resemble those seen after administration of a progestogen.

The antiestrogen tamoxifen, may, when endogenous estrogen levels are low, act as an estrogen and endometrial proliferative activity may

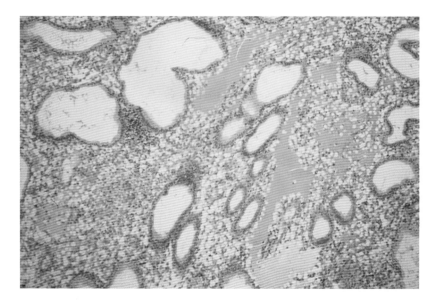

Figure 4.10. Irregular glandular ripening in luteal phase insufficiency: the glands to the upper left are dilated by secretion and of normal appearance for the mid-secretory phase but those to the lower right are narrow and weakly secretory or inactive

be seen. Its use may also be complicated by the development of polyps and, rarely, malignancy (see below).

Biopsy diagnosis of functional endometrial abnormalities

The biopsy diagnosis of functional endometrial abnormalities is dependent upon the receipt of a representative tissue sample of adequate size accompanied by a full clinical and menstrual history. Endometrial samples sent for histopathological assessment may be unrepresentative if there are, for example, underlying leiomyomas, causing thinning of the endometrium, and may be too small for a full assessment if they consist only of superficial fragments. Interpretation may also be hindered if the pathologist is not told the day of the cycle on which the biopsy was taken or does not have the full details of the woman's hormone therapy or therapeutic drug usage. Drugs may upset the pituitary–ovarian hormone control; the latter may include antidepressants.

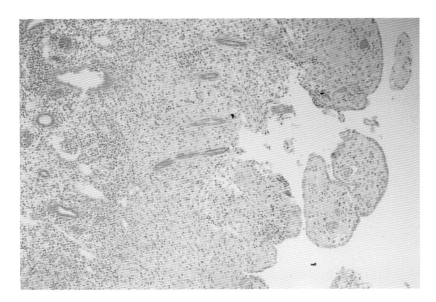

Figure 4.11. The endometrial contact site of a progestogen-impregnated contraceptive device; note the pseudodecidual stromal change, the narrow inactive glands and the papillary surface

Inflammation and infection in the endometrium

The endometrium normally contains a population of lymphocytes and, at the time of menstruation, polymorphonuclear leucocytes. The presence of such cells in the endometrium is therefore not indicative of an inflammatory process. Plasma cells, eosinophils, tissue breakdown associated with a polymorphonuclear leucocyte infiltrate at times other than at menstruation, granulomas and lymphoid aggregates with germinal centres are, however, not normally found in the endometrium and are regarded as hallmarks of inflammation.

NON-INFECTIVE INFLAMMATION

Inflammation which is not infective in origin may be physiological, such as that which accompanies the remodelling of the decidua in the early stages of pregnancy or following delivery, or it may be pathological. The latter type occurs when there is abnormal tissue breakdown in the uterine cavity; for example, when there is torsion of a polyp, in association with an intrauterine contraceptive device, when there is prolonged and frequent heavy bleeding or in the presence of a neoplasm.

INFECTION OF THE ENDOMETRIUM

Endometrial infections are uncommon because the establishment of an infective lesion is discouraged by the efficient downward drainage of the uterine cavity, the regular shedding of the endometrium in the reproductive years and the presence of an effective cervical mucus barrier that prevents the ascent of most organisms into the uterus from the cervix and vagina.

If, however, these natural protective mechanisms are disturbed, endometritis may supervene. Thus, drainage from the uterine cavity may be partly or completely obstructed by polyps, neoplasms or retained products of conception within the uterine cavity, by acute flexion of the uterus, by scarring of the cervix following surgery, obstetric trauma or radiotherapy or by a cervical neoplasm. Disruption of the cervical mucus barrier occurs in women:

- with chronic cervical infection, in whom mucus secretion may be impaired

- in whom previous cervical surgery has removed much of the mucus-secreting tissue

- who have had operative procedures involving dilatation or biopsy of the cervix.

The mucus barrier does not offer complete protection, as certain organisms such as *Neisseria gonorrhoeae* are capable of penetrating it. Interruption of endometrial shedding, for reasons other than pregnancy, does not in itself predispose to infection but permits any infection that may occur to become established. The uterus has little natural protection against those infections which spread via the bloodstream or descend from the fallopian tubes.

Pathological features of endometrial inflammation

Inflammation may be acute, subacute or chronic and chronic inflammatory lesions may be granulomatous or non-granulomatous. Acute endometritis is recognised by the presence, in the endometrium, of polymorphonuclear leucocytes associated with tissue destruction at times other than at menstruation. Acute infections are usually poly-microbial and occur most commonly following miscarriage, although an acute endometritis may be caused by gonococcal infection.

In active chronic endometrial inflammation (Figure 4.12) plasma cells, polymorphonuclear leucocytes, lymphocytes and histiocytes are found in the stroma and polymorphonuclear leucocytes are present in the glandular lumens. If inflammation is particularly severe, there may be disturbances in the induction of hormone receptors, as a consequence of which the tissue may fail to reflect the normal cyclical hormonal changes.

The incidence of chronic non-granulomatous endometritis is difficult to determine and is almost certainly underestimated because of the difficulty in distinguishing an abnormal diffuse chronic inflammatory cell infiltrate from the normal lymphocytic population of the endometrium. The presence of lymphoid follicles with germinal centres is, however, always abnormal. When the inflammatory infiltrate is predominantly histiocytic the term histiocytic or xanthomatous endometritis is sometimes used (Figure 4.13).

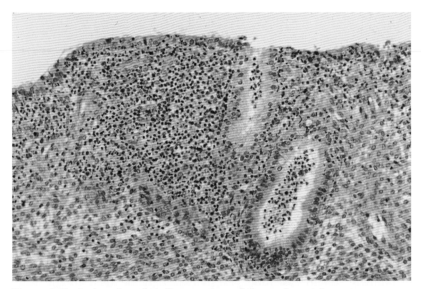

Figure 4.12. Active chronic inflammation of the endometrium at an intrauterine contraceptive device contact site: the stroma is heavily infiltrated by polymorphs, plasma cells and lymphocytes and the gland contains an acute inflammatory cell infiltrate (reproduced with permission from Buckley and Fox, *Biopsy Pathology of the Endometrium,* 2nd ed., published by Edward Arnold)

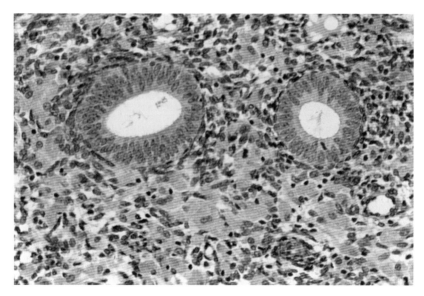

Figure 4.13. Non-specific chronic inflammation of the endometrium: the stroma is infiltrated by lymphocytes and large, pink-staining, histiocytes; occasional plasma cells are present: this appearance may be termed histiocytic or xanthomatous endometritis

Chronic granulomatous inflammation in the endometrium is regarded as being caused by tuberculosis until otherwise proven and, indeed, non-tuberculous granulomatous inflammation is extremely uncommon. Endometrial tuberculosis is almost always secondary to infection in the fallopian tubes, from which site there is repeated inoculation of the endometrial surface. The regular menstrual shedding of the endometrium tends to prevent establishment of infection and, because the shedding of the endometrium occurs at about the same interval as the time taken for a granuloma to be recognisable histologically, granulomas tend to be small and poorly developed (Figure 4.14). Caseation is rarely seen unless endometrial shedding has been incomplete, when caseating granulomas may be seen in the basal endometrium or after the menopause, when extensive, confluent, caseating endometrial tuberculosis may be encountered. The presence of intraluminal neutrophil polymorphonuclear leucocytes may be the only histological abnormality in tuberculous infection of the endometrium.

Consequences of endometrial inflammation

Acute inflammation has no long-term adverse effects unless infection persists, there is secondary infection or infection spreads to the fallopian tubes. When inflammation is so severe that there is structural damage to the basal layers of the endometrium, tissue regrowth may be hampered, a condition known as Asherman syndrome. When this happens, the stroma may be extensively replaced by fibrous tissue, intrauterine adhesions may be formed and the glands may be unresponsive to normal hormonal stimulation. Similar changes may develop after endometrial resection.

Endometrial metaplasia

The tissue of the müllerian system (that is, the fallopian tubes, uterus and endocervix) retain into adulthood a capacity to differentiate into one or more of the tissues to which the paracoelomic epithelium, the embryonic precursor of the müllerian tract, gives rise during fetal development. In the adult, this takes the form of epithelial metaplasia which, in the endometrium, is usually characterised by replacement of the epithelial lining of one or more glands, completely or partly, by a squamous (Figure 4.15), serous (Figure 4.16) or mucinous (Figure 4.17) epithelium. This is most common in hyperestrogenic states and in elderly postmenopausal women. In older women with cervical obstruction and intrauterine infection, the uterus may become lined only by squamous epithelium, a condition known as 'ichthyosis uteri' and one which may occasionally give rise to a squamous cell carcinoma. Focal intraglandular squamous metaplasia also occurs in adenocarcinomas of the endometrium and is discussed below. Endometrial stromal metaplasia, with bone, cartilage or smooth muscle formation, also occurs but is extremely uncommon.

Endometrial polyps

The term 'endometrial polyp' could be used to describe any polypoidal lesion protruding into the uterine cavity. By convention, however, the term is restricted to non-neoplastic pedunculated or sessile nodules composed of either functional or basal endometrium or a combination of the two. Endometrial polyps develop as a consequence of focal stromal and glandular overgrowth. It is believed that focal hypersensitivity to estrogen or lack of sensitivity to progesterone may allow a portion of endometrium to remain unshed at the end of menstruation. This focus continues to grow in each successive cycle until it protrudes into the uterine cavity. Polyps of distinctive histological appearance are also found

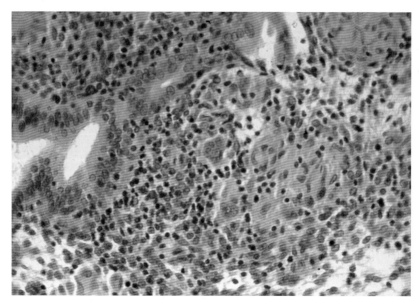

Figure 4.14. Endometrial tuberculosis: a very early, poorly developed, noncaseating granuloma lies in the stroma (to the lower right); it is composed of epithelioid macrophages and lymphocytes

in women taking tamoxifen. Polyps do not occur before the menarche. They are most common in the fifth decade of life and are sometimes encountered in postmenopausal women.

Endometrial polyps vary greatly, ranging from small lesions discovered incidentally to large masses which protrude from the cervical os. They may be sessile or pedunculated. In the reproductive years, they are usually composed either of non-functional basal endometrium or they have a central core of basal-type endometrium containing thick-walled arteries covered by a layer of functional endometrium of variable thickness. The latter is frequently out of step with the endometrium elsewhere in the uterine cavity; for example, showing only weak proliferative activity during the follicular phase and either lacking secretory features or showing only weak or patchy secretory activity in the luteal phase. The tip of the polyp is often congested, even to the naked eye, and focally inflamed. Ulceration may occur and the surface epithelium may undergo squamous metaplasia, this being seen particularly in those polyps protruding from the cervical os or developing from the uterine isthmus. On rare occasions, pedun-

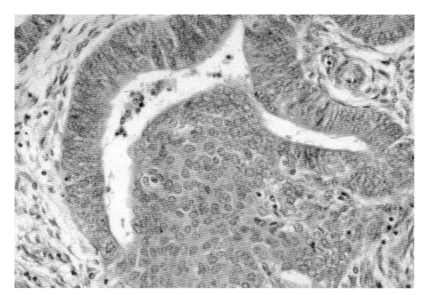

Figure 4.15. Intraglandular squamous metaplasia of the endometrium: a focus of bland metaplastic squamous epithelium replaces part of the lining of this hyperplastic endometrial gland and protrudes into the lumen

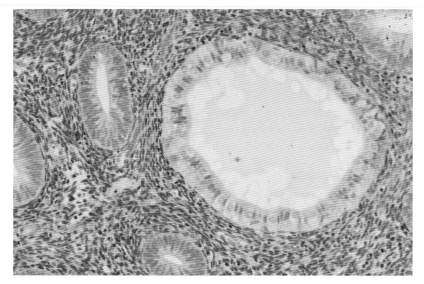

Figure 4.16. Serous or tubal metaplasia of the endometrium in a single gland in the centre of the field: the other glands are lined by an inactive, postmenopausal epithelium

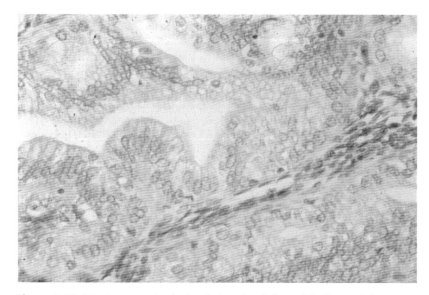

Figure 4.17. Mucinous metaplasia of the glandular epithelium of the endometrium

culated polyps may undergo torsion and infarction. Polyps in postmenopausal women may be formed either of inactive basal-type endometrium or of cystically atrophic endometrium with a fibrous stroma (Figure 4.18).

Polyps commonly recur, presumably because they have been incompletely removed or because the underlying defect persists. Polyps do not predispose to the development of a carcinoma. Malignant change occasionally occurs in polyps but most apparent instances of this phenomenon have actually been adenocarcinomas growing in a polypoidal fashion. The exception to this is the development of malignancy in polyps associated with long-term use of tamoxifen.

Specific forms of polyp which require special mention include those in which the stroma, although partially or largely of endometrial type, also contains bands of smooth muscle. These comprise the adenomyomatous polyp and the atypical polypoid adenomyoma (Figure 4.19), which is characterised by glandular architectural and cytological atypia. The latter are benign but may be confused in biopsy specimens with endometrioid adenocarcinoma and there may be, on very rare occasions, adenocarcinomatous change within them.

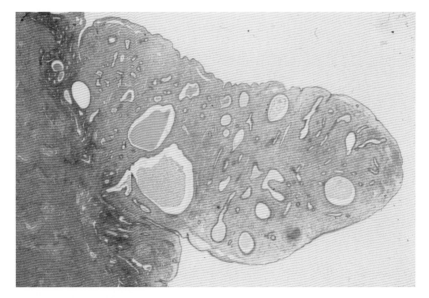

Figure 4.18. An endometrial polyp: this is composed of endometrial tissue in which some of the glands are cystically dilated and the stroma more fibrous than the adjacent nonpolypoidal endometrium which is inactive; this is a postmenopausal lesion

Endometrial hyperplasia

Endometrial hyperplasia is widely regarded as a possible precursor of endometrial adenocarcinoma. The term 'endometrial hyperplasia' encompasses, however, several distinct conditions and it is important to distinguish between those types of hyperplasia associated with a significant risk of evolving into an adenocarcinoma and those devoid of any such risk (Figure 4.20). The defining feature of an endometrial hyperplasia indicative of a propensity for malignant change is cytological atypia. Any hyperplastic lesion of the endometrium showing this abnormality is classed as 'atypical hyperplasia'. Hyperplastic conditions that lack cytological atypia are divided into 'simple' and 'complex' forms. The biological factors that determine the type of hyperplastic response of the endometrium are unknown.

SIMPLE ENDOMETRIAL HYPERPLASIA

Simple hyperplasia (also often but incorrectly called cystic glandular hyperplasia) is a relatively common condition. It represents the physiological response of the endometrium to prolonged, unopposed

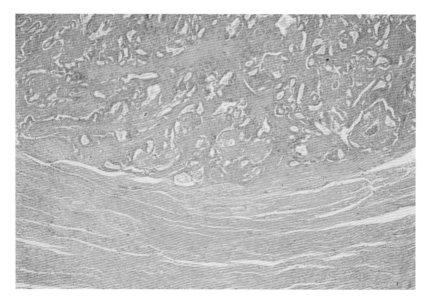

Figure 4.19. An atypical polypoid adenomyoma: this is composed of glands of variable shape and size set in a stroma in which there is smooth muscle; note the well-defined margin at the junction with the underlying myometrium

estrogenic stimulation, being in fact only one component of a general-ised hyperplasia of all the uterine tissues. The endometrium is thickened and often polypoidal. The entire endometrium is involved and there is a loss of the normal distinction between basal and functional zones. The endometrial glands show a proliferative pattern but vary markedly in calibre, some being unusually wide, others of normal calibre and yet others unduly narrow (Figure 4.21). The glandular epithelium is formed by plump cuboidal or low columnar cells with basophilic cytoplasm and round, centrally or basally situated nuclei. The endometrial stroma shares in the hyperplastic process and hence the gland-to-stroma ratio is normal with no glandular crowding. The stroma appears hypercellular while mitotic figures, present in both glands and stroma, may be sparse or abundant but are invariably of normal form. Foci of adenomyosis and endometriosis are also affected.

Simple hyperplasia may complicate exogenous estrogen therapy, estrogenic ovarian tumours or polycystic ovary syndrome. The most common cause of the condition is, however, a series of anovulatory cycles in which estrogen production by persistent ovarian follicles is not opposed

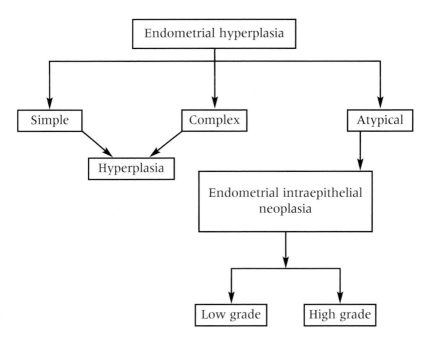

Figure 4.20. Classification of endometrial hyperplasia

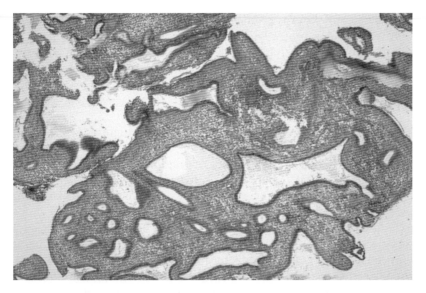

Figure 4.21. Simple endometrial hyperplasia: the endometrium contains glands of varying calibre, some being normal and others being cystically dilated

by any luteal secretion of progesterone. Hence, this type of hyperplasia occurs most commonly in the perimenarchal and perimenopausal years, when anovulatory cycles are common. If ovulatory cycles are resumed or if progestogen is administered, simple hyperplasia will regress and the endometrium will rapidly return to its normal state.

Simple endometrial hyperplasia alone is not a precursor of, and does not evolve into, atypical endometrial hyperplasia and is not associated with any increased risk of developing an adenocarcinoma.

COMPLEX HYPERPLASIA

Complex hyperplasia may occur under the same circumstances as simple hyperplasia: that is, in an endometrium exposed to unopposed estrogenic stimulation, but it can also develop in a normally cycling or atrophic endometrium. A complex hyperplasia is restricted to the glandular component of the endometrium and does not involve the stroma. It is usually focal or multifocal in nature, involving only a group or groups of glands. The hyperplastic glands are variable in size, often larger than normal, and are crowded together with a reduction in the amount of intervening stroma. The involved glands show an abnormal pattern of growth with outpouchings or buddings of the glandular epithelium into the stroma to give a 'finger-in-glove' pattern (Figure 4.22). Intraluminal epithelial tufting is also common. The glandular epithelium is regular and formed of cuboidal or columnar cells with basal or central nuclei and there is no cytological atypia. The risk of a complex hyperplasia evolving into an adenocarcinoma has not been fully determined but is almost certainly extremely low.

ATYPICAL HYPERPLASIA

Atypical hyperplasia develops under the same circumstances as does complex hyperplasia, some cases being 'estrogen driven' and others apparently occurring in the absence of undue estrogenic stimulation of the endometrium. As with complex hyperplasia, only the glands are hyperplastic and the lesions are either focal or multifocal. In the hyperplastic areas (Figure 4.23), there is crowding of the glands with a marked reduction in intervening stroma. In severe cases, the glands show a 'back-to-back' pattern, the stroma between the glands being reduced to a thin wisp or completely obliterated. The glands are usually irregular in shape and are lined with cells showing varying degrees of atypia. In milder forms of atypical hyperplasia, the epithelial nuclei tend to be ovoid with retention of polarity and of a near normal chromatin pattern, however much the nucleocytoplasmic ratio has

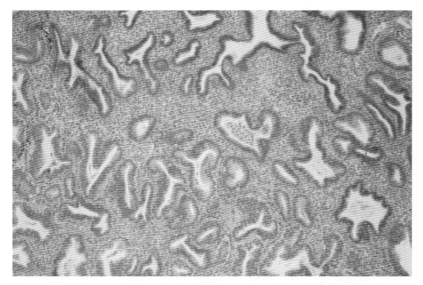

Figure 4.22. Complex hyperplasia of the endometrium: the endometrial glands are more closely packed than normal and irregular in outline (reproduced with permission from Buckley and Fox, *Biopsy Pathology of the Endometrium*, 2nd ed., published by Edward Arnold)

increased. In more severe cases, the nuclei are round and enlarged, nuclear polarity is lost, nucleoli are increased in size and there is an abnormal chromatin pattern. With progressing severity of atypia, there is an increasing degree of epithelial multilayering and of intraluminal tufting.

Atypical hyperplasia can undoubtedly evolve into endometrial adenocarcinoma. The exact magnitude of this risk is not adequately defined but a reasonable estimate would be that approximately 25% of cases of atypical endometrial hyperplasia will eventually give rise to an invasive endometrial adenocarcinoma. When considering this progression from an atypical hyperplasia to an invasive neoplasm, it is widely assumed that the controlled proliferation of a hyperplastic process may 'slip over' into the cellular anarchy of neoplasia. It must be doubted, however, whether this is a viable concept and there are good grounds for believing that the lesion classed as an atypical hyperplasia of the endometrium is a form of endometrial intraepithelial neoplasia, comparable in many respects to CIN or CGIN. The fact that many cases of atypical hyperplasia will regress if treated with a progestogen does not conflict with this hypothesis.

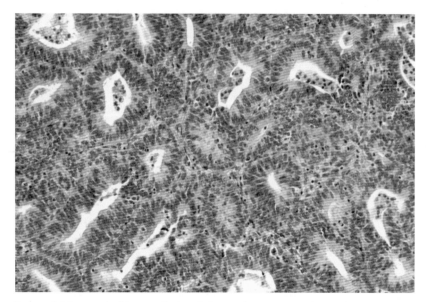

Figure 4.23. Atypical hyperplasia of the endometrium: the endometrial glands are closely packed and lined by an epithelium in which there is cellular stratification, nuclear enlargement and hyperchromasia

More suitable nomenclature than 'atypical hyperplasia' has therefore been proposed. Suggested terms include 'intraendometrial neoplasia', on the assumption that it may be impossible, particularly in biopsy specimens, to distinguish carcinomas limited to the endometrium from non-invasive lesions; 'endometrial intraepithelial neoplasia', on the assumption that the pathologist can, with certainty distinguish an intraepithelial abnormality from a carcinoma limited to the endometrium; and endometrioid neoplasia. Of these terms, 'intraendometrial neoplasia' appears to be the most satisfactory (Figure 4.20).

Serous endometrial intraepithelial carcinoma (Figure 4.24) is a concomitant of, or putative precursor of serous carcinoma. It therefore has a more serious implication (see below) and should not be confused with endometrial intraepithelial neoplasia. These lesions overexpress p53 as do many serous carcinomas. The realisation that many cases of apparent serous endometrial intraepithelial carcinoma are, in fact, associated with extrauterine malignancy questions the validity of serous endometrial intraepithelial carcinoma as a distinct entity.

Malignant epithelial tumours of the endometrium

The vast majority of endometrial neoplasms are adenocarcinomas, which develop most commonly during the sixth decade, many women being in the early postmenopausal years. Only about 5% of these neoplasms occur in premenopausal women. It is traditionally maintained that women who develop endometrial adenocarcinoma are commonly nulliparous, often have an unusually late menopause and have a high incidence of hypertension, diabetes mellitus and obesity. The association of this neoplasm with nulliparity and a late menopause has withstood the test of case–control studies but there is considerable doubt as to whether there is any direct link with either hypertension or diabetes. It is certain, however, that obese women have a significantly increased risk of developing endometrial adenocarcinoma.

ENDOMETRIOID ADENOCARCINOMA

The role of estrogens in the pathogenesis of endometrial adenocarcinoma has been much debated but it is now well established that the administration of exogenous estrogens is associated with a greatly

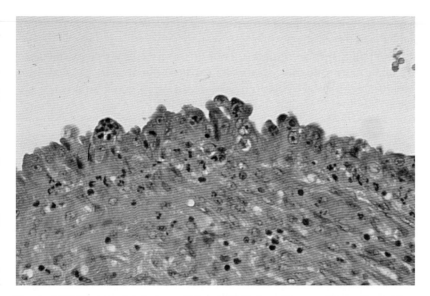

Figure 4.24. Endometrial serous intraepithelial carcinoma: the surface of the endometrium is covered by a layer of focally budding, highly atypical cells with large pleomorphic nuclei and large irregular nucleoli

increased risk of developing endometrioid endometrial adenocarcinoma. In the USA, the rise of incidence of this neoplasm, which occurred after the introduction of widespread unopposed estrogen hormonal replacement therapy, was rapid. This suggests that, under these circumstances, estrogens were acting as a promoter substance, exposure to a presumed initiator mechanism being therefore common. It is thus established that estrogens can be implicated in the pathogenesis of some endometrial adenocarcinomas. It remains uncertain, however, whether an overproduction of endogenous estrogen is of aetiological importance in those women who form the vast majority of cases and who develop endometrial adenocarcinoma in the absence of exogenous hormones. It is certainly true that women with estrogen-secreting ovarian tumours have a notably high incidence of associated endometrial adenocarcinoma but such cases represent only a tiny minority. Many women with endometrial adenocarcinoma have, however, an increased ability to convert androstenedione, of adrenal origin, into estrone. This conversion occurs principally by aromatase in the fat cells of the body and this is probably why obese women, with their excess number of fat cells, are particularly prone to develop endometrial neoplasia. A similar estrone excess would, of course, result as a consequence of a primary overproduction of androstenedione and it is therefore of particular note that women with untreated polycystic ovary syndrome, in which there is excessive ovarian synthesis of androstenedione, suffer not only a high incidence of adenocarcinoma but tend to develop the neoplasm at an unusually early age (characteristically in their late twenties).

Even taking into account the above factors, it is clear that by no means all endometrial adenocarcinomas are estrogen-related. A significant proportion of these neoplasms arise in an atrophic endometrium and these are probably not estrogen-driven. The pathogenesis of such tumours is obscure but it is of note that they often appear to be more aggressive than are those which occur in a setting of hyperestrogenism.

An endometrial adenocarcinoma may appear as a localised plaque, polyp or nodule, usually in the upper part of the uterus. More commonly, the tumour presents as a diffuse nodular or polypoidal thickening of the uterine lining or as a bulky friable mass which fills or even distends the uterine cavity.

Histologically, most endometrial adenocarcinomas show a greater or lesser degree of endometrial differentiation and are classed as 'endometrioid adenocarcinomas'. Many are well differentiated (histological grade 1) and bear a resemblance, albeit an anarchic one, to normal proliferative endometrium (Figure 4.25). They are formed of irregular, tightly packed, convoluted glandular acini lined by columnar cells showing a variable degree of pleomorphism, nuclear hyper-

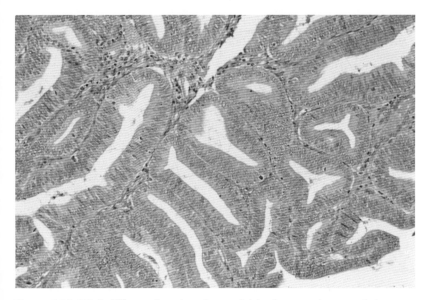

Figure 4.25. Well-differentiated endometrioid adenocarcinoma of the endometrium: the tumour is composed of closely packed, well-formed glands lined by stratified cells with enlarged nuclei; mitoses are present

chromatism and mitotic activity, commonly with irregular multi-layering and intraluminal tufting. The stroma is scanty and in many cases obliterated. Foci of necrosis, haemorrhage and leucocytic infiltration are common and there may be a noteworthy accumulation of foamy stromal histiocytes. Less well-differentiated endometrioid adenocarcinomas (histological grades 2 and 3) grow in a more solid fashion and grading of these neoplasms is based upon a consideration of both the proportion of the tumour showing a solid growth pattern and the degree of cytological atypia (Table 4.1).

Most endometrioid adenocarcinomas contain foci of bland squamous metaplasia but, even if widespread, this does not alter the prognosis for any given adenocarcinoma. Uncommitted cells in the endometrium may also differentiate along endocervical lines and thus give rise to the rare mucinous adenocarcinoma of the endometrium. Small areas of mucinous differentiation are often found in endometrioid adeno-carcinomas but their presence does not affect the outcome. A diagnosis of mucinous adenocarcinoma is made if the mucinous component of the neoplasm exceeds 30%.

Well-differentiated endometrioid adenocarcinomas tend to be slowly growing. They often remain within the confines of the uterus for a considerable time, spreading initially by direct invasion of the

Table 4.1 Grading of endometrial carcinoma

ARCHITECTURAL GRADING OF ENDOMETRIOID CARCINOMA (Modified from FIGO)	
Grade 1	5% or less of the tumour shows a solid growth pattern
Grade 2	Between 5% and 50% of the tumour is growing in a solid pattern
Grade 3	More than 50% of the tumour shows a solid growth pattern. Notable nuclear atypia inappropriate for the architectural grade, raises the grade of a grade 1 or 2 tumour by one grade

CYTOLOGICAL GRADING OF ENDOMETRIOID CARCINOMA (After Zaino *et al.* 1995)	
Grade 1	Rounded to oval nuclei with evenly distributed chromatin and inconspicuous nucleoli
Grade 2	Irregular oval nuclei with chromatin clumping and moderate sized nucleoli
Grade 3	Large pleomorphic nuclei with coarse chromatin and large irregular nucleoli

myometrium and cervix. Later, the neoplasm may penetrate the uterine serosa and seed into the pouch of Douglas and on to the pelvic peritoneum. Cornual carcinomas commonly extend into the fallopian tubes and tumour cells may pass through the tubal ostia to be deposited on the ovaries and pelvic peritoneum. Local spread may also involve the broad ligament and the parametrium. Lymphatic spread occurs to pelvic and para-aortic nodes, while haematogenous dissemination to lungs, liver, adrenals and bones occurs late. It should be stressed that this slow pattern of growth is only a feature of well-differentiated endometrioid tumours.

A further point of some importance is that tumours arising from a background of atypical hyperplasia have a better prognosis than do those developing in an atrophic endometrium. The overall 5-year survival for women with endometrial adenocarcinoma is about 65%. Stage is clearly of prognostic importance (Table 4.2) but other features related to survival are the grade of the neoplasm and the histological type, serous tumours and clear-cell adenocarcinomas having a poor prognosis. Other prognostic factors to be taken into account are those indicative of a poor outlook:

- deep invasion of the myometrium
- the presence of tumour cells in vascular spaces
- a lack of estrogen and progesterone receptors
- an aneuploid DNA pattern.

Table 4.2. Staging of endometrial carcinoma (FIGO)

Stage		Description
I		**Tumour is confined to the corpus uteri**
	Ia	Tumour is confined to the endometrium
	Ib	Tumour invades the inner half of the myometrium
	Ic	Tumour extends into the outer half of the myometrium
II		**Tumour involves the corpus and cervix**
	IIa	Tumour involves the endocervical glands
	IIb	Tumour involves the cervical stroma
III		**Tumour extends outside the uterus but not outside the true pelvis**
	IIIa	Tumour extends through the serosa to the adnexa, or there are positive peritoneal washings
	IIIb	Tumour involves the vagina
	IIIc	Tumour involves peritoneal or pelvic lymph nodes
IV		**Tumour extends beyond the true pelvis or has involved the mucosa of the bladder or rectum**
	IVa	Tumour involves the bladder or rectal mucosa
	IVb	Tumour has metastasised to distant sites, including abdominal or inguinal lymph nodes

SEROUS ADENOCARCINOMA

Serous carcinomas (Figure 4.26) histologically resemble a tubal adeno-carcinoma and they frequently develop in an atrophic endometrium. The whole tumour may show serous differentiation or serous carcinoma may form part of a neoplasm that is predominantly endometrioid or contains areas of clear-cell differentiation. Serous carcinomas are high-grade neoplasms and are all regarded as histological grade 3, the nuclear grade taking precedence over the architectural features and the presence of serous carcinoma taking precedence over any endometrioid component. The tumours generally overexpress p53 as a consequence of mutation of the *p53* gene. At the time of diagnosis, even when of relatively low volume, they have frequently spread into the vasculature of the uterus and disseminated widely. Neoplasms of this type may arise from uncommitted müllerian cells which pursue a tubal, rather than an endometrial, pathway of differentiation.

CLEAR-CELL CARCINOMA

Clear-cell adenocarcinomas, identical histologically to clear-cell neoplasms of the vagina and ovary (Figure 4.27), also occur in the endometrium. Areas of serous carcinoma may coexist and clear-cell carcinoma areas may

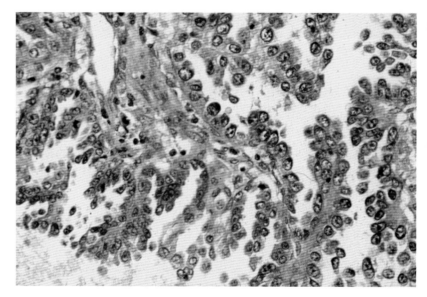

Figure 4.26. Serous adenocarcinoma of the endometrium: the tumour is composed of papillae covered by cells of serous or tubal type, which are poorly differentiated and have large nuclei with high nucleocytoplasmic ratios

develop in endometrioid adenocarcinomas. The neoplasms are all regarded as high grade and nuclear grading takes precedence over architectural differentiation: they are, therefore, histological grade 3.

Both serous and clear-cell carcinomas pursue an aggressive course, with early, deep penetration of the myometrium, sometimes striking microscopic intravascular and intralymphatic permeation and spread to para-aortic nodes.

ADENOSQUAMOUS CARCINOMA

Adenosquamous carcinomas account for about 5% of endometrial neoplasms. They contain an admixture of both adenocarcinoma and squamous cell carcinoma (Figure 4.28). They differ from an adeno-carcinoma with squamous metaplasia in so far as the squamous tissue is clearly malignant and invasive. Adenosquamous carcinomas tend to occur at a relatively late age and run an aggressive course, the 5-year survival rate being below 40%.

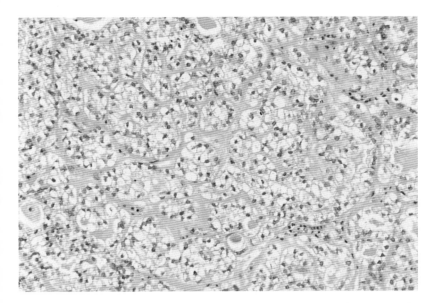

Figure 4.27. Clear-cell adenocarcinoma of the endometrium: the tumour is composed of cells with well-demarcated margins, large nuclei and copious clear cytoplasm

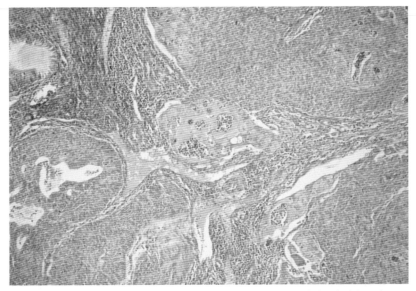

Figure 4.28. Adenosquamous carcinoma: in the centre of the field and to the upper right, there is focally keratinising squamous cell carcinoma; to the lower left, there is variably differentiated adenocarcinoma

SQUAMOUS CELL CARCINOMA

The endometrium is a rare site for squamous cell carcinoma. This type of neoplasm usually develops in elderly women with pyometra and complete squamous metaplasia of the surface epithelium (ichthyosis uteri). In younger women, CIN may spread upwards into the uterine body, where it replaces the surface epithelium and can give rise to a squamous cell carcinoma. The prognosis for a squamous cell carcinoma of the endometrium is extremely poor.

UNDIFFERENTIATED CARCINOMA

Undifferentiated carcinomas show no evidence of glandular or specific epithelial differentiation and can be differentiated from lymphomas, neuroendocrine tumours and sarcomas only by the presence of epithelial markers. They have a poor prognosis.

SMALL-CELL CARCINOMA

Small-cell neuroendocrine tumours occur in postmenopausal women and are histologically identical to bronchial small-cell carcinomas. Foci of such tumour may occur admixed with endometrioid adenocarcinoma. They have a poor prognosis. They are distinct from primitive neuroectodermal tumours, which are exceedingly rare in the endometrium.

Malignant stromal tumours of the endometrium

ENDOMETRIAL STROMAL SARCOMA

Endometrial stromal sarcomas are formed of cells which resemble those of the endometrial stroma during the proliferative phase of the menstrual cycle. These neoplasms have traditionally been divided into low-grade and high-grade types, this distinction being based upon mitotic counts. It is now accepted, however, that most tumours classed as high-grade stromal sarcomas do not contain endometrial stromal-like cells and should be classed as undifferentiated uterine sarcomas. Furthermore, in cases that do meet the diagnostic criteria for an endometrial stromal neoplasm, mitotic counts are of no prognostic value and so the distinction between high-grade and low-grade endometrial stromal sarcomas is no longer valid. Some stromal sarcomas contain a minor degree of epithelial differentiation, others have a so-called sex cord pattern; some contain small smooth muscle elements and others show rhabdoid differentiation. These features do not appear to affect the outcome. It is important to recognise the so-called 'stromal nodule' which is also composed of endometrial stromal-like tissue but is benign.

Endometrial stromal sarcomas can form localised tumour masses but they have a particular tendency to infiltrate the vascular and lymphatic channels of the myometrium extensively. Cords of tumour tissue may therefore protrude from the cut surface of the uterus, giving it a 'comedo' or 'rough towel' appearance. Histologically (Figure 4.29), the neoplasms are formed of sheets of spindle-shaped cells, which resemble the endometrial stromal cells of the normal proliferative phase. The cells contain progesterone receptors. Endometrial stromal sarcomas run an indolently malignant course. They tend to spread into the parametrium and often recur locally, sometimes as long as 20 years after removal of the primary tumour. Approximately 20% of women with these neoplasms will eventually succumb, usually after an extremely protracted course.

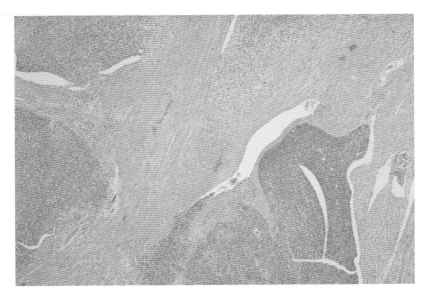

Figure 4.29. An endometrial stromal sarcoma of the uterus: the vascular spaces of the myometrium are permeated by a tumour composed of fairly regular uniform cells resembling those of the normal endometrial stroma

SMOOTH MUSCLE TUMOURS

Small leiomyomas contained within and limited to the endometrium may occasionally be encountered. More commonly, however, they have their primary origin in the myometrium and come to lie in a submucous site.

Mixed tumours of the endometrium

Although most endometrial neoplasms are either purely epithelial or solely mesenchymal, a few show a bimorphic pattern and contain both epithelial and non-epithelial tissues. Such neoplasms, often classed as 'mixed müllerian tumours', may be of low-grade malignancy and contain a benign epithelial component and a malignant mesenchymal element (adenosarcomas) or can be of high-grade malignancy with both epithelial and mesenchymal elements being malignant (carcinosarcoma). The epithelial component of a mixed tumour is usually of a type normally found in the müllerian system but, although the mesenchymal component commonly differentiates into either smooth muscle or endometrial stromal-like cells (that is, into tissues which are homologous for the uterus), it can also differentiate into tissue normally alien to the uterus, the most common of such heterologous elements being striated muscle, bone and cartilage.

Mixed tumours of high-grade malignancy, carcinosarcomas, are of unknown aetiology. They occur principally in elderly women and form bulky, fleshy polypoid masses which fill the uterine cavity, sometimes extending into the endocervical canal and occasionally protruding through to the vagina. Histologically, they consist of an intimate admixture of carcinomatous and sarcomatous tissues (Figure 4.30). The adenocarcinomatous element usually resembles an endometrioid adenocarcinoma and the sarcomatous element is either undifferentiated or resembles an endometrial stromal sarcoma. Heterologous tissues may be present (Figure 4.31) but these are of no diagnostic or prognostic significance.

Endometrial carcinosarcomas are highly aggressive neoplasms which tend to spread rapidly outside the uterus and metastasise via the bloodstream, the prognosis being generally poor. The most important prognostic factor for these neoplasms, apart from stage, is the grade of the carcinomatous component. This fact, together with molecular findings, has led to the belief that carcinosarcomas are 'metaplastic carcinomas' or 'sarcomatoid carcinomas'.

Mixed tumours of low-grade malignancy, adenosarcomas, resemble carcinosarcomas macroscopically but have a benign epithelial

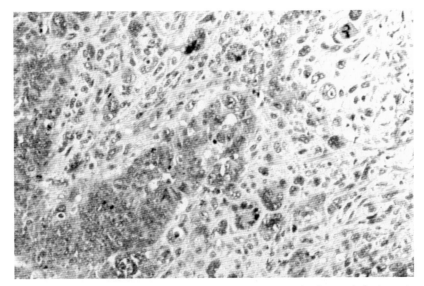

Figure 4.30. Carcinosarcoma of the endometrium: to the lower left there is poorly differentiated adenocarcinoma and to the right there is spindle-celled sarcomatous tissue containing some multinucleated cells with large darkly staining nuclei

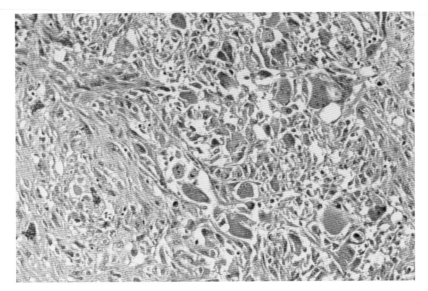

Figure 4.31. Carcinosarcoma of the endometrium with heterologous elements: in this sarcomatous area, the large cells with copious pink cytoplasm are rhabdomyoblasts

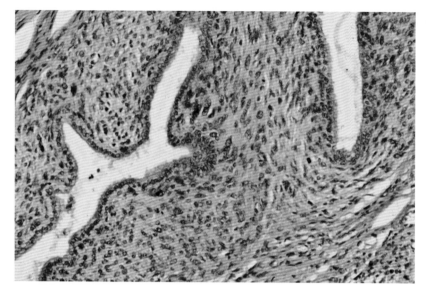

Figure 4.32. Adenosarcoma of the endometrium: the glands are lined by a benign neoplastic epithelium of cervical and endometrial type and the periglandular stroma is composed of cells with large, hyperchromatic, pleomorphic nuclei

component, of endometrial, endocervical or tubal type, set in a stroma resembling an endometrial stromal sarcoma (Figure 4.32). Heterologous elements may be present. The neoplasms spread outside the uterus in only about 50% of cases and distant metastases are very uncommon. Even women with spread outside the uterus (but limited to the pelvis) may survive for prolonged periods as this tumour pursues an indolently malignant course.

5 The myometrium

Non-neoplastic conditions of the myometrium

ADENOMYOSIS

Adenomyosis is characterised by the presence of endometrial tissue deep within the myometrium and there is almost invariably an associated hypertrophy of smooth muscle around the ectopic islands of endometrium. The foci of endometrial tissue may be distributed diffusely within the myometrium, in which case the uterus shows a roughly symmetrical enlargement, or can be focal, forming a poorly-defined tumour-like asymmetrical thickening of the myometrium (Figure 5.1). The localised form is often known as an 'adenomyoma', an unfortunate term because of its misleading connotation of neoplasia. Histologically, foci of adenomyosis consist of both endometrial glands and stroma (Figure 5.2). The glands are usually of basal type and thus do not show cyclic activity.

Adenomyosis is caused by a downgrowth of basal endometrium into the myometrium. Serial sectioning shows continuity between the basal endometrium and foci of adenomyosis. The aetiology of this diverticular disease is, however, obscure, for although both curettage and estrogenic stimulation have been proposed as aetiological factors, there is no proof that either is of causal significance.

VASCULITIS

The majority of cases of vasculitis of the myometrium are isolated lesions, particularly when they affect only the small vessels. Occasionally, however, larger arteries are affected and the possibility of there being a systemic arteritis should be considered.

INFLAMMATION

Infection in the endometrium may spread to the myometrium following childbirth, miscarriage or intrauterine surgery. On rare occasions, however, non-infective inflammation may develop in systemic disease, such as sarcoidosis (Figure 5.3).

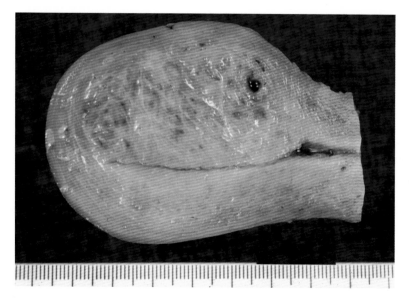

Figure 5.1. Adenomyosis: there is an asymmetrical thickening of the uterine wall; islands of focal haemorrhage can be seen among the hypertrophied muscle (reproduced with permission from McGee JO, Isaacson PG, Wright NA, editors. *Oxford Textbook of Pathology*, published by Oxford University Press)

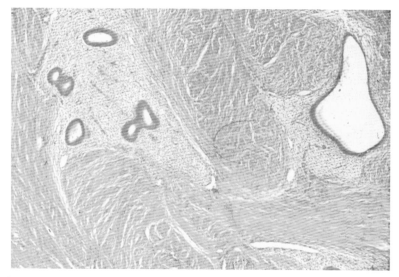

Figure 5.2. Adenomyosis: within the myometrium there are islands of endometrial tissue of basal type which contain glands and stroma (reproduced with permission from Fox and Buckley, *Atlas of Gynaecological Pathology*, published by MTP Press)

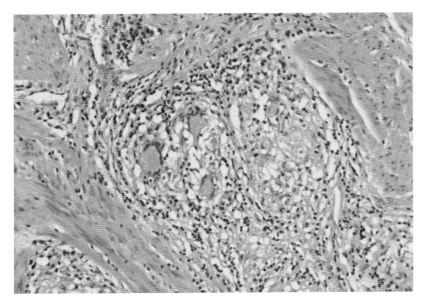

Figure 5.3. Sarcoidosis in the myometrium: a well-formed, noncaseating epithelioid granuloma, in which there are three giant cells, lies between the muscle fibres

Benign tumours

LEIOMYOMAS

Leiomyomas are tumours of the smooth muscle cells of the myometrium. There is commonly an intermingling with fibrous tissue and the tumours are often inaccurately known as 'fibroids'. Myometrial leiomyomas are extremely common, being present in at least 25% of women above the age of 35 years and there is considerable circumstantial evidence that estrogenic stimulation plays a role in their pathogenesis. Consequently, they develop only during the reproductive years, enlarge both during pregnancy and in women using contraceptive steroids and tend to shrink after the menopause.

The tumours are usually multiple and vary in size from tiny 'seedlings' to huge masses which fill the abdomen. They may be within the uterine wall (intramural), in a submucosal site immediately below the endometrium or may lie just below the peritoneal covering of the uterus in a subserosal site. Submucosal leiomyomas tend to bulge into and distort the uterine cavity, with thinning of the overlying endometrium. They sometimes become polypoid to form a mass which may fill the uterine cavity and can also extend through the endocervical canal into the vagina. Subserosal tumours may grow out from the uterine surface and can extend into the broad ligament. They may also become pedunculated. Such a neoplasm may, in rare cases, become attached to the omentum or pelvic peritoneum where, after losing its stalk, it derives a new blood supply and flourishes as a parasitic leiomyoma.

Uterine leiomyomas have a well-defined regular outline with a surrounding pseudocapsule of compressed muscle fibres. When sectioned, they have a firm, bulging, white, whorled or trabeculated appearance. Histologically, they consist of smooth muscle fibres arranged in bundles and whorls (Figure 5.4). The cells are elongated with spindle- or cigar-shaped nuclei. Some tumours, known as cellular leiomyomas, contain densely-packed cells with elongated nuclei. Rarely, the smooth muscle cells are rounded with central nuclei and clear cytoplasm. Tumours containing such cells are classed as epithelioid leiomyomas. Other variants of the usual pattern include the neurilemmoma-like leiomyoma, in which the nuclei show a pallisaded pattern; the symplastic leiomyoma (Figure 5.5), characterised by the presence of bizarre multinucleated cells, and the mitotically active leiomyoma showing no other features of malignancy (Table 5.1).

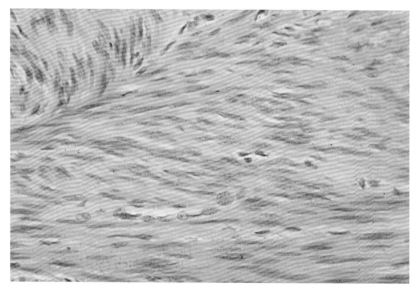

Figure 5.4. Uterine leiomyoma: the tumour is composed of interweaving bands of elongated smooth muscle cells; no mitotic figures are present

Table 5.1. Smooth muscle tumours of the uterus

	Mitotically active	Bizarre/ symplastic	Sarcoma
Well-defined margin	Yes	Yes	No
Haemorrhage	No	No	Yes
Necrosis	Possibly	Possibly	Yes
Cellularity	Yes	Possibly	Yes
Increased mitoses	Yes	No	Yes
Cellular pleomorphism	No	Yes	Yes
Associated with hormonal therapy	Yes	Yes	No

In all but the smallest leiomyomas, degenerative changes tend to occur, owing to the neoplasm outgrowing its blood supply. Consequently, hyaline change, cystic change, myxoid degeneration, patchy necrosis and calcification are common. A pedunculated submucosal tumour may undergo torsion and infarction. A specific form of necrosis, seen particularly but not only in pregnancy, is 'red degeneration' (Figure 5.6),

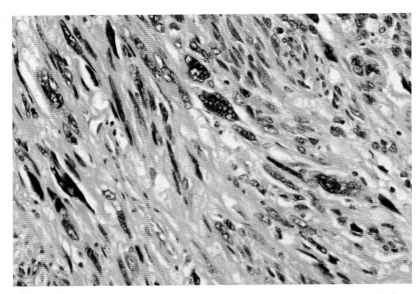

Figure 5.5. Symplastic or bizarre leiomyoma: the tumour is composed of interweaving bands of elongated smooth muscle cells in which the nuclei vary in size, are enlarged and darkly staining; no mitotic figures are present

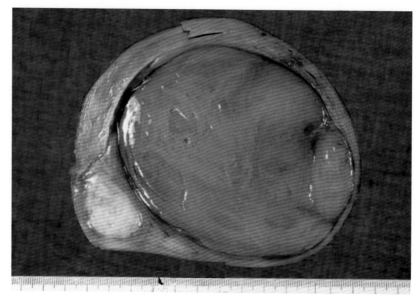

Figure 5.6. Red degeneration of a leiomyoma: the uterus is distorted by a large, dusky red-coloured leiomyoma which has lost its normal trabecular pattern; this contrasts with the smaller leiomyoma of usual appearance to the lower left

characterised by a dull, beefy red appearance of the tumour, which may also have a slightly fishy odour. This change can be accompanied by pain and fever. The presence of thrombosed vessels suggests that it represents haemorrhagic infarction of an extensively hyalinised neoplasm.

Malignant change very rarely occurs in uterine leiomyomas. However, certain variants of a leiomyoma, although histologically benign, do appear to behave in an invasive fashion. Thus, in the condition of 'intravenous leiomyomatosis' cords of smooth muscle are found in uterine and parauterine veins, usually in association with more conventional leiomyomas elsewhere in the myometrium. The plugs of tumour cells occasionally extend as far as the inferior vena cava and can grow into the right atrium. It is not clear whether this condition is a special form of leiomyoma which, despite its benign nature, invades veins, or whether the tumours arise from the vein walls. A not dissimilar condition is benign metastasising leiomyoma, in which histologically benign uterine leiomyomas appear to be associated with pulmonary metastases which show no malignant features. Such cases probably represent the simultaneous independent development of pulmonary and uterine leiomyomas. In disseminated peritoneal

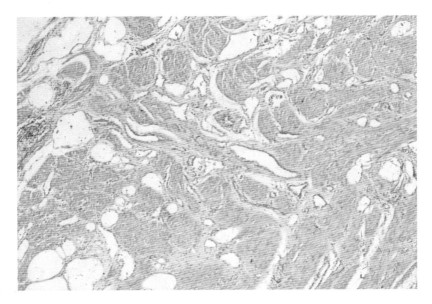

Figure 5.7. Adenomatoid tumour of the myometrium: cystic spaces lined by flattened epithelium form a honeycomb which replaces much of the outer third of the myometrium (reproduced with permission from Fox and Buckley, *Atlas of Gynaecological Pathology*, published by MTP Press)

leiomyomatosis, small leiomyomatous nodules are found scattered in the peritoneum and omentum in association with uterine leiomyomas. It is thought, however, that these extrauterine nodules arise in situ from the submesothelial mesenchyme of the peritoneum.

OTHER BENIGN TUMOURS

Fibromas, lipomas and haemangiomas can all occur in the myometrium but the only other benign myometrial neoplasm which is not of extreme rarity is the adenomatoid tumour. Neoplasms of this type are present in 1% of uteri and appear as small, rather poorly-delineated, masses in the cornual region, usually in an immediately subserosal site. Histologically (Figure 5.7), they are formed of complex multiple gland-like spaces which are lined by flattened or low cuboidal cells and are separated from each other by strands of fibromuscular tissue. Adenomatoid tumours are benign, almost invariably asymptomatic and are derived from the serosa, having all the characteristics of a benign mesothelioma.

Atypical polypoid leiomyoma is discussed in Chapter 4.

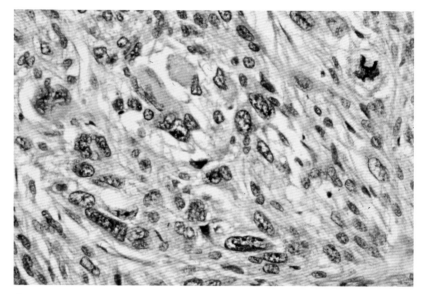

Figure 5.8. Leiomyosarcoma of the uterus: the tumour is composed of cells which vary in size and shape, several being multinucleated; an atypical mitosis (lies to the upper right)

Malignant neoplasms

LEIOMYOSARCOMA

These are rare, accounting for only 1% of malignant uterine neoplasms, and occur most commonly in the fifth and sixth decades of life (Table 5.1). The tumours are less well demarcated than are leiomyomas. They often show areas of haemorrhage or necrosis and are characterised histologically by their cellularity, pleomorphism and high mitotic counts (Figure 5.8). Myometrial leiomyosarcomas spread locally to invade the pelvic organs but it is uncommon for lymph node metastases to occur. However, blood-borne spread to the lungs, liver and kidneys is common. The 5-year survival rate for women with a neoplasm of this type is only 20–30%.

METASTATIC TUMOURS

Lymphomas may infiltrate the uterus, diffusely enlarging the uterus and the appendages or producing a local mass. Metastatic carcinomas in the myometrium usually have a primary origin in the genital tract

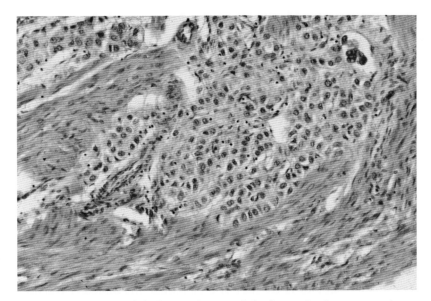

Figure 5.9. Metastatic lobular carcinoma of the breast in the myometrium: the tumours cells are of regular size and infiltrate between the muscle bundles of the myometrium

but, occasionally, metastases from the stomach, colon or breast (Figure 5.9) may be limited to the myometrium. Metastases from other extragenital sites occur much more rarely.

6 The fallopian tube and broad ligament

Inflammation of the fallopian tube

Inflammation of the fallopian tube (salpingitis) is a common disorder of the reproductive years. It is almost invariably infective, although minor degrees of irritative inflammation may occur as a response to the presence of necrotic tissue or blood in the tube due to, for example, menstrual reflux, bleeding from endometriotic foci or the presence of an ectopic gestation. There may also be a mild inflammatory response to foreign bodies, such as those used in sterilisation procedures.

It is difficult to determine accurately the true incidence of infective salpingitis as most cases are not confirmed either histologically or bacteriologically at the time they present and depend only upon clinical criteria for their diagnosis, particularly in the acute phase.

The term 'pelvic inflammatory disease' (PID) is used to encompass signs and symptoms caused by inflammation centred on the fallopian tube but extending, in many cases, to involve the ovary, mesosalpinx, parametrium, uterine serosa and uterine ligaments. In the acute phase, the clinical features are of an acute febrile illness associated with pelvic pain, vaginal discharge and tenderness over the fallopian tube. Chronic or subacute salpingitis may be recognised only when investigations for infertility are undertaken, this being a common complication of the disorder. It should be emphasised that the term PID refers only to a clinical concept and is one that should not be used as a pathological diagnosis.

Infection reaches the tube by one of three routes. Most commonly, infection ascends from the lower genital tract along the mucosal surface of the tube, causing an endosalpingitis. Less commonly, it may spread via the lymphatics to the wall of the tube from the uterus or other adjacent organs, causing an interstitial salpingitis. Least commonly, infection may be blood-borne. The inflammation may be non-granulomatous or granulomatous, the former being much more common.

ASCENDING INFECTION

Infection that spreads from the uterine cavity along the mucosal surface of the uterus and fallopian tube is characteristic of, for example, *Neisseria gonorrhoeae*, chlamydial infection and infection associated with the presence of an intrauterine contraceptive device but many cases are of a non-specific polymicrobial nature.

In an acute endosalpingitis the tube is tense and swollen, the serosa congested and the subserosal tissues oedematous. In severe infections, the serosa may be covered by a fibrinous exudate. The mucosa is oedematous, hyperaemic and focally haemorrhagic. The lumen contains pus which may leak from the ostium and the fimbria, as they become inflamed and 'sticky', tend to undergo agglutination and invagination until, finally, the ostium may be occluded. In ascending infections, as might be expected, the mucosa bears the brunt of the damage.

The oedematous tubal plicae are infiltrated by polymorphonuclear leucocytes and the lumen contains an acute inflammatory exudate and tissue debris (Figure 6.1). In severe infections, there is mucosal ulceration and the inflammatory infiltrate may extend through the wall to the peritoneum, causing a local peritonitis. In repeated or chronic infections, plasma cells, lymphocytes and histiocytes predominate; the

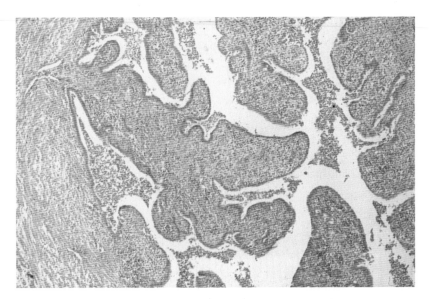

Figure 6.1. Acute endosalpingitis: the mucosal folds are oedematous and are infiltrated by acute inflammatory cells; the lumen contains a purulent exudate

latter may, in long-standing cases, be the main cell type. If inflammation subsides rapidly or is only mild, there may be little or no residual tubal damage but unfortunately an attack of salpingitis predisposes to further attacks. Full recovery becomes progressively less likely with each succeeding episode and the risk of permanent damage, leading to infertility or ectopic pregnancy, more certain.

Severe inflammation may be complicated by local or generalised peritonitis, extension of infection to the adjacent ovary, the development of a tubo-ovarian abscess or a pelvic abscess. Systemic dissemination of infection can occur, particularly in gonococcal infections, and may cause an arthritis or endocarditis. Repeated attacks of acute endosalpingitis may lead to the development of a pyosalpinx (a pus-filled fallopian tube) (Figure 6.2) in which there is usually extensive ulceration of the mucosa. Such a severe degree of damage is irrecoverable.

Long-term sequelae of endosalpingitis may be minimal and limited to minor fibrous scars in the mucosa or the musculature, or they may be major. As the ulcerated mucosa, particularly in the ampulla, heals there may be fusion of the plical folds across the lumen of the tube to produce a mesh, this being known as follicular salpingitis (Figure 6.3). Plical fusion of this type may also be seen in a tube which is, in

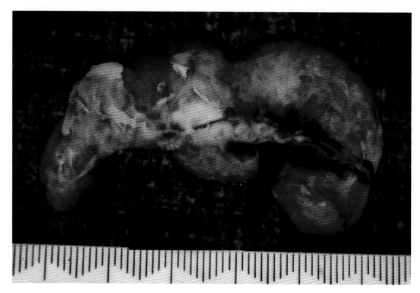

Figure 6.2. Pyosalpinx: the fallopian tube is swollen, reddened and the serosa is covered by a fibrinous exudate; the fimbria are invaginated and the ostium is occluded

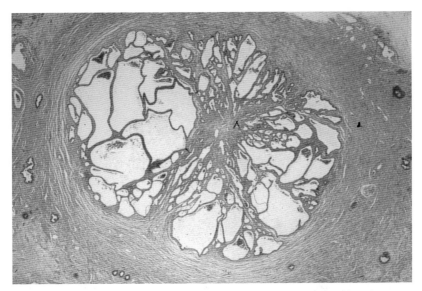

Figure 6.3. Follicular salpingitis: the plicae are extensively fused to form a honeycomb-like mesh across the tubal lumen: there is no active inflammation (reproduced with permission from McGee JO, Isaacson PG, Wright NA, editors. *Oxford Textbook of Pathology*, published by Oxford University Press)

addition, distended by clear watery fluid and in which the ostium is occluded, a condition known as a follicular hydrosalpinx. A hydrosalpinx may also occur in the absence of mucosal fold fusion and in such cases the tube assumes a retort shape and the wall is thin and translucent with the mucosa characteristically intact but rather flattened (Figure 6.4). Conversely, after prolonged or severe tubal inflammation, the tube may be thick-walled and rather rigid as a consequence of intramural and subserosal fibrosis.

Changes may also occur in the isthmus as a consequence of damage, usually associated with some degree of obstruction in the outer part of the tube. Diverticula, associated with muscular hypertrophy, develop in the isthmus, a condition known as 'salpingitis isthmica nodosa' because of the nodules which can be seen or felt in the wall of the isthmus (Figure 6.5). This condition appears to be secondary to an increase in intraluminal pressure and is, in our experience, not encountered when the remainder of the tube is normal. It is not, as has been previously suggested, a direct, but rather an indirect effect of inflammation.

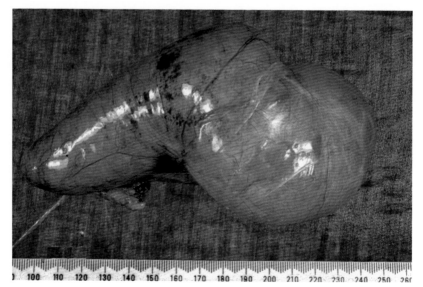

Figure 6.4. Hydrosalpinx: the distension of the fallopian tube is maximal in the ampulla creating a retort-like shape; the tube wall is thin and translucent

LYMPHATIC INFECTION

Lymphatic infection classically follows postpartum or postabortive infection and is uncommon today. The interstitial tissues of the tube are the main focus of the inflammatory assault, with relative sparing of the tubal mucosa. As a consequence, the lumen may remain patent and mechanical obstruction of the tube is an unlikely outcome. However, inflammation is rarely limited to the tube wall and it is usual to find a coexisting endosalpingitis.

BLOOD-BORNE INFECTION

Blood-borne infection is typified by tuberculosis which, although it may spread directly to the tube from the peritoneal cavity, urinary tract or gastrointestinal tract or via the lymphatics from the intestinal tract, is more likely to arise as a consequence of blood-borne infection from a distant focus. At the time of diagnosis, the tube has often become converted into a retort-shaped, fibrotic sac which may be focally calcified and contain caseous material. Classically, the tubal ostium

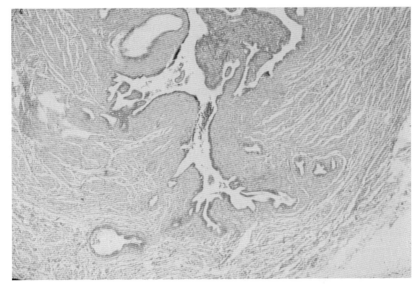

Figure 6.5. Salpingitis isthmica nodosa: diverticular disease of the fallopian tube; there are glandular spaces in the musculature of the wall which are continuous with the lumen in the upper part of the field (reproduced with permission from Fox and Buckley, *Pathology for Gynaecologists*, 2nd ed., published by Edward Arnold)

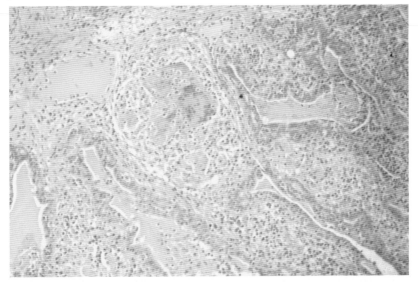

Figure 6.6. Tuberculosis of the fallopian tube: there is a noncaseating, sarcoid-like, epithelioid granuloma, containing Langerhans giant cells, in the centre of the field; the mucosal folds are swollen and infiltrated by chronic inflammatory cells and the lumen is distended by fluid

remains patent and the fimbria relatively normal. Histological examination (Figure 6.6) shows a chronic endosalpingitis with caseating, or non-caseating, intramucosal granulomas, the latter more closely resembling sarcoid-like granulomas than the tuberculous granulomas encountered in tuberculosis elsewhere in the body. In long-standing disease, the tube may be lined only by focally calcified fibrous tissue in which it may be difficult to find specific tubercular features.

In some parts of the world, schistosomiasis is endemic and the condition is sometimes encountered in women who have visited East Africa. The parasitic eggs may be found in any of the pelvic organs where they elicit a granulomatous inflammatory response (Figure 6.7).

DIRECT SPREAD OF INFLAMMATION TO THE TUBE

The situation of the tube within the pelvis means that it will inevitably be involved by infection of other pelvic organs when there is local peritonitis. It may, therefore, be affected by appendicitis or diverticular disease of the large bowel. It may also be involved in systemic diseases such as Crohn's disease (Figure 6.8).

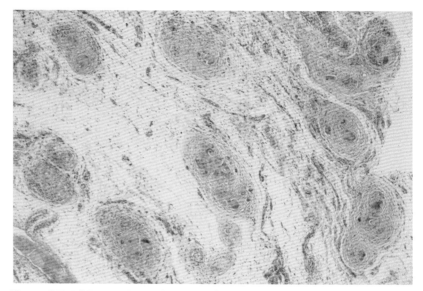

Figure 6.7. Schistosomiasis: the paratubal tissue contains numerous granulomas which have developed around the ova of the parasites

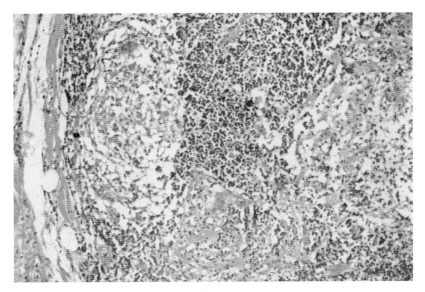

Figure 6.8. Crohn's disease of the fallopian tube: the tube wall contains several ill-defined granulomas among a diffuse lymphocytic infiltrate (reproduced with permission from Fox and Buckley, *Atlas of Gynaecological Pathology*, published by MTP Press)

Cysts

A variety of cysts are commonly found in the tissues surrounding the fallopian tube. The majority develop in müllerian duct remnants (paramesonephric cysts) or wolffian duct remnants (mesonephric cysts). Only rarely, for example when they undergo torsion or reach an unusually large size, do they become clinically apparent. The majority of these cysts are thin-walled, often translucent, and may be pedunculated. Those of müllerian origin, which include the extremely common hydatid of Morgagni, which is pedunculated and attached to the fimbria, are lined by epithelium of tubal type (Figure 6.9). Those of wolffian origin are lined by a single layer of cubocolumnar cells. Their walls are fibrous and those of paramesonephric origin tend to contain more muscle than do those of müllerian origin. On rare occasions, epithelial neoplasms may develop within these cysts (Figure 6.10).

The tubal serosa commonly exhibits focal transitional or uroepithelial metaplasia (so-called Walthard's rests) (Figure 6.11), which may also undergo cystic change. They rarely become more than a few millimetres in diameter and appear as yellow-grey specks or pinhead-size granules on the serosal surface of the tube.

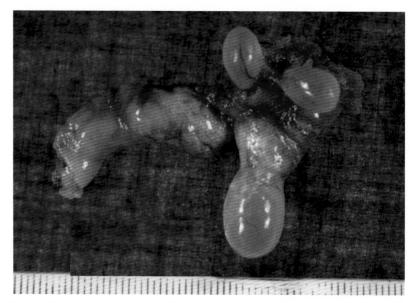

Figure 6.9. Fimbrial cysts: the fimbrial end of the tube bears several, small, thin-walled cysts

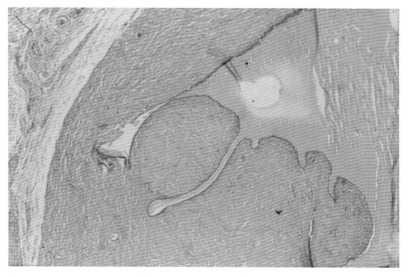

Figure 6.10. Serous adenofibroma arising within a paratubal cyst: arising from the cyst wall is a serous tumour with coarse, fibrous papillae (reproduced with permission from Fox and Buckley, *Atlas of Gynaecological Pathology*, published by MTP Press)

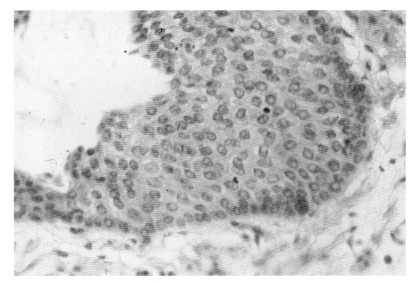

Figure 6.11. Cystic Walthard's rest: the cyst is lined by uroepithelium

Tumours of the fallopian tube

Neoplasms of the fallopian tube are rare. Carcinomas, which are the most common tumours, constitute only 0.3% of malignant gynae-cological neoplasms.

BENIGN NEOPLASMS

Benign intraluminal epithelial tumours of the tube may be sessile or polypoidal and typically form small adenofibromas. In the interstitial segment of the tube, they are usually of endometrial type whereas, in the remainder of the tube, they have a fibrous stroma and the epithelium is of tubal type.

Adenomatoid tumours, which are of mesothelial origin, may develop in the tubal lumen but more commonly grow eccentrically in a subserosal site, locally invaginating the tube wall. They appear as small, usually not exceeding 1–2 cm, round to ovoid, firm, grey to yellow-white, well-circumscribed nodules. Histologically (Figure 6.12), they are composed of tubules and gland-like spaces lined by flattened cuboidal cells set in a fibrous stroma and are not encapsulated.

Other very rare benign neoplasms of the fallopian tube include lipomas, which are generally subserosal, leiomyomas, fibromas,

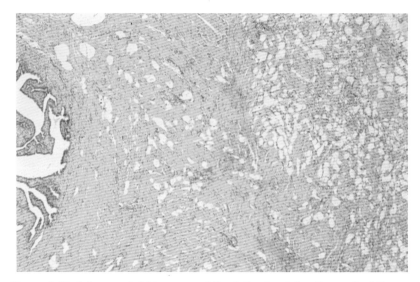

Figure 6.12. Adenomatoid tumour of the fallopian tube: the wall of the tube is infiltrated by small, tightly packed, glandular spaces, some of which are cystic; they are most numerous in the subserosal area, to the right

haemangiomas and neurilemmomas. Mature cystic teratomas have also, exceptionally, been described in the fallopian tube.

MALIGNANT NEOPLASMS

The most common primary malignant neoplasms are adenocarcinomas. Most cases occur in older women, the average age being in the sixth decade of life. Some tumours are associated with mutations of the *BRCA1* and *BRCA2* genes with which ovarian and breast cancers are also associated.

The majority of tumours are unilateral and 10–20% are bilateral. The lesion starts as a small plaque, nodule or polypoidal lesion within the lumen (Figure 6.13), most commonly at the junction of the middle and outer thirds of the tube but usually by the time of diagnosis the tube is distended by tumour. The tube becomes retort-shaped and grossly resembles a hydrosalpinx or pyosalpinx but, unless there has been preceding inflammation, it is usual for the fimbria to be normal and the ostium patent. It is unusual for a tumour to have penetrated the wall of the tube. In a small minority of cases, the tumour is confined to the fimbrial portion of the tube.

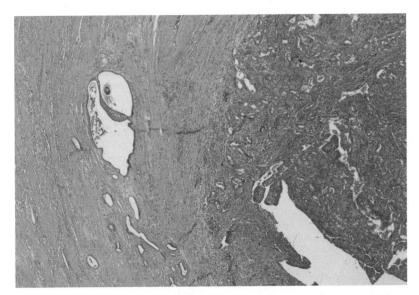

Figure 6.13. Adenocarcinoma of the fallopian tube: a small, polypoidal carcinoma protrudes into the lumen of the tube, to the right

Most carcinomas are well-differentiated papillary adenocarcinomas that closely resemble serous carcinomas of the ovary. Less well-differentiated tumours have a mixed alveolar–papillary pattern and the least well-differentiated neoplasms tend to grow in a solid fashion. Endometrioid and transitional cell tumours also occur. The tumour spreads directly via the tubal ostium to the peritoneum; via the uterine ostium into the uterus and directly through the tube wall to the adjacent structures. Lymphatic spread occurs to the uterus, ovary and the iliac and para-aortic lymph nodes. The late presentation of the tumours means that the average survival at 5 years for women with a tubal carcinoma is only about 15%. Further, it is unusual for a diagnosis of tubal carcinoma to be made prior to surgery.

Tubal carcinomas have to be distinguished clinically and histologically from tumours that have metastasised or spread to the tube, for example from the ovary or uterus (Figure 6.14), and which are more common than primary neoplasms. Such a distinction is facilitated by identifying an area of carcinoma in situ within the residual tubal epithelium (Figure 6.15), from which the carcinoma can be seen to arise. In many cases a distinction may be impossible. Nevertheless, there is a growing awareness that some apparent primary serous adenocarcinomas of the ovary or peritoneum are actually primary tumours of the fallopian tube.

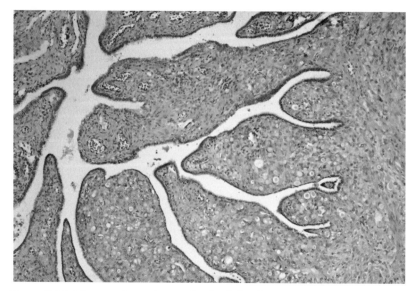

Figure 6.14. Metastatic carcinoma in the fallopian tube: the mucosal folds are expanded by infiltrating lobular carcinoma of the breast

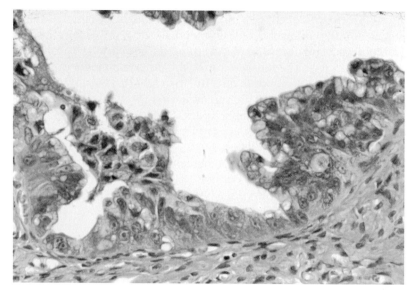

Figure 6.15. Adenocarcinoma in situ of the fallopian tube: the epithelium is stratified and composed of cells with large pleomorphic nuclei in which there are large irregular nucleoli

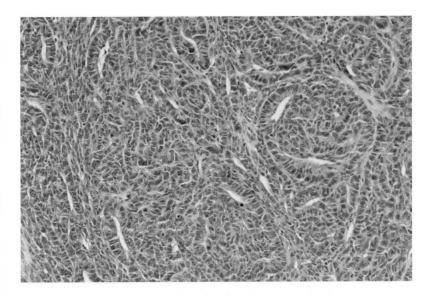

Figure 6.16. Adnexal tumour of probable wolffian origin: the tumour is composed of tubules and trabeculae set in a scanty fibrous stroma

Tumours of the broad ligament

Benign tumours of the broad ligament are rare, with the exception of leiomyomas, which resemble those occurring in other sites. Many so-called broad ligament leiomyomas actually have their origin from the outer surface of the myometrium and grow into the broad ligament.

Serous neoplasms (see above) may develop in paratubal cysts and these may be benign, borderline or malignant, the latter being exceptionally rare.

A tumour specific to this site is the female adnexal tumour of probable wolffian origin, although some studies have suggested an origin from the rete ovarii. The tumour is generally benign but, exceptionally, may behave in a malignant fashion. Tumours are solid or solid and cystic and vary in size up to 25 cm. They lie within the broad ligament or within the subserosa of the fallopian tube. Histologically, they vary in appearance; tubules, cysts or trabeculae are set in a fibrous stroma (Figure 6.16). Immunohistochemistry has suggested an origin from the rete ovarii rather than wolffian duct remnants.

Malignant tumours of the broad ligament are more likely to be metastatic than of primary origin.

7 The ovary

Inflammation

NON-INFECTIVE INFLAMMATION

Non-infective inflammation is not common but may occur as a response to bleeding from endometriotic foci. It is also seen in ovaries that have undergone torsion. A granulomatous inflammatory response may occur owing to starch granules from surgical gloves, keratin derived from ruptured mature cystic teratomas or hysterosalpingographic contrast material (Figure 7.1).

INFECTIVE INFLAMMATION

Most infections of the ovary are non-specific in nature and polymicrobial in origin. Infection may be caused by blood-borne infection from remote foci. In the acute phase, the ovary is reddened and oedematous. A polymorphonuclear infiltrate is present in the superficial cortex and there may be a fibrinous exudate on the ovarian surface (Figure 7.2). It is rare for infection to extend deeply into the ovary but when it does there may be abscess formation (Figure 7.3). The chronic phase is characterised by fibrosis of the ovarian surface epithelium and the formation of periovarian adhesions (Figure 7.4).

Non-neoplastic cysts

Non-neoplastic cysts of the ovary may develop from the surface epithelium, follicles, endometriotic foci or may occasionally be the end result of an abscess. Most are asymptomatic, whatever their origin, but some become clinically apparent because of their large size, by undergoing torsion or their hormonal activity.

CYSTS DERIVED FROM THE SURFACE EPITHELIUM

The most common cysts derived from the surface epithelium are the

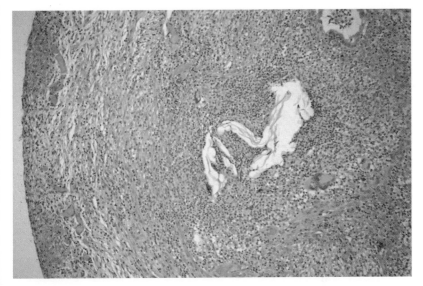

Figure 7.1. Foreign body granuloma in the ovarian cortex elicited by keratin from a ruptured mature teratoma

hormonally inactive epithelial or serous inclusion cysts (Figure 7.5) which develop as a consequence of invagination of the surface epithelium of the ovary into the stroma, particularly at the site of ovulation. The invaginations lose their connection with the surface epithelium and, because of secretion of fluid, become cystic. These cysts may be single or multiple and can occur at any age. They may lie deep or superficially in the cortex and vary in size from a few millimetres to several centimetres. By convention, although perhaps illogically and incorrectly, cysts measuring more than 3 cm in diameter are classed as benign serous cystadenomas. The epithelium lining the cysts is usually tubal in nature but may, less commonly, be endometrioid or endocervical in type.

CYSTS DERIVED FROM THE FOLLICLES

Follicular cysts are common but those measuring less than 2.5 cm in diameter are regarded as being physiological and are classed as cystic follicles rather than as follicular cysts. Within this definition, follicular cysts are usually single, although multiple cysts of this type are encountered in the ovarian hyperstimulation and polycystic ovary syndromes.

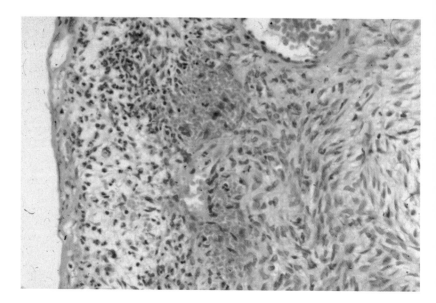

Figure 7.2. Acute inflammation of the ovary: the blood vessels in the cortex are dilated and there is a neutrophil polymorphonuclear cell infiltrate

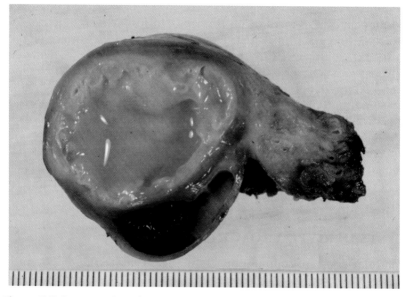

Figure 7.3. Intraovarian abscess: the abscess cavity contains purulent material and the blood vessels in the surrounding ovarian tissue are dilated producing a red rim

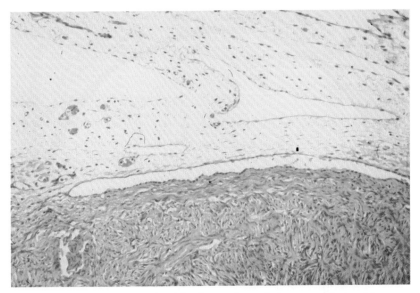

Figure 7.4. Chronic perioophoritis: the surface of the ovary (below) is covered by fine, delicate fibrovascular connective tissue adhesions

Solitary follicular cysts can occur at any age and are thin-walled and unilocular. They range in size from 3 cm to 10 cm (Figure 7.6) and are lined by an inner layer of granulosa cells and an outer layer of thecal cells. Most follicular cysts are asymptomatic but some appear to be estrogenic and are associated with symptoms such as precocious puberty, menstrual disturbances or, after the menopause, postmenopausal bleeding (Figure 7.7). Occasionally, a follicular cyst may rupture and cause a haemoperitoneum. Solitary follicular cysts may develop during pregnancy and can achieve a very large size (Figure 7.8).

Corpus luteum cysts (Figure 7.9) are again distinguished from a cystic corpus luteum by their size. Cysts of this type have a convoluted lining of large luteinised granulosa cells and smaller luteinised thecal cells with an innermost layer of fibrous tissue. Such cysts probably occur when the central cavity of a ruptured follicle is unusually large or when there is excessive intrafollicular haemorrhage at the time of ovulation.

OVARIAN HYPERSTIMULATION SYNDROME

This condition is characterised by the presence of multiple theca–lutein cysts in the ovaries which are usually bilateral and may cause considerable ovarian enlargement (Figure 7.10). The cysts are of

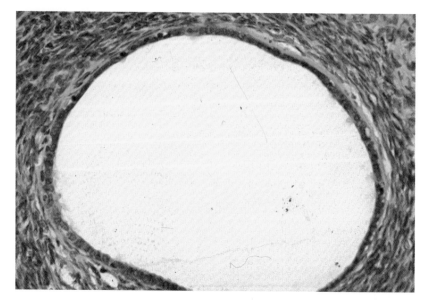

Figure 7.5. Epithelial inclusion cyst: the cyst, within the ovarian cortex is lined by a single layer of epithelium of serous type

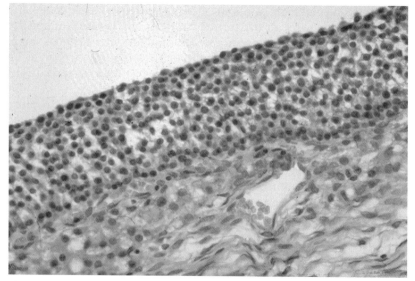

Figure 7.6. Follicular cyst of the ovary: the cyst is lined by a broad band of uniform granulosa cells with regular darkly staining nuclei: the larger, paler cells of the theca interna lie deep to the granulosa cells (reproduced with permission from Fox and Buckley, *Atlas of Gynaecological Pathology*, published by MTP Press)

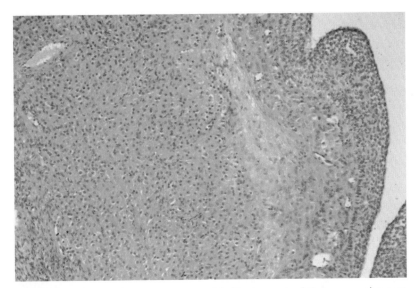

Figure 7.7. Luteinised postmenopausal follicular cyst of the ovary: the cyst is lined by luteinised granulosa cells and the thecal cells in the wall are also heavily luteinised

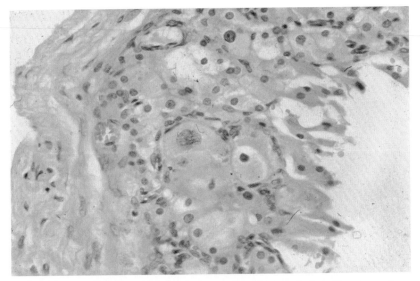

Figure 7.8. Giant follicular cyst of pregnancy: the cyst is lined by several layers of heavily luteinised pleomorphic granulosa cells (reproduced with permission from Fox and Buckley, *Atlas of Gynaecological Pathology*, published by MTP Press)

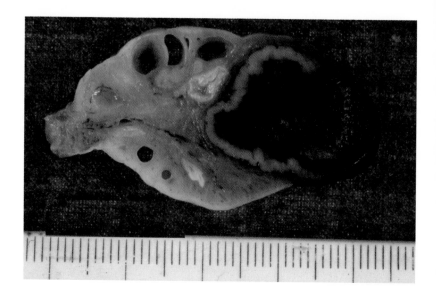

Figure 7.9. Haemorrhagic corpus luteum cyst of the ovary: the cyst, to the right, has a yellow wall and contains blood

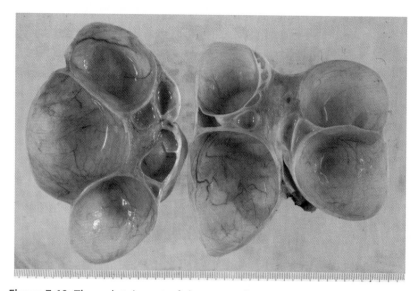

Figure 7.10. Theca–lutein cyst of the ovary: the ovaries are enlarged by the presence of several, thin-walled, theca–lutein cysts

follicular origin but have a lining in which the theca interna cells are hyperplastic and heavily luteinised with granulosa cells being either absent or markedly luteinised. Cysts of this type are caused by excessive stimulation of the ovary by human chorionic gonadotrophin (hCG) and may occur in:

● normal pregnancy

● multiple pregnancy

● women with hydatidiform mole or choriocarcinoma

● women undergoing artificial stimulation of the ovary as part of the treatment of infertility.

There is an increased tendency for ovaries containing multiple theca–lutein cysts to undergo torsion and the woman may present with abdominal pain. Some women become mildly virilised because of production of androgens by the theca–lutein cysts and ascites is occasionally encountered. The cysts usually regress after removal of their cause.

POLYCYSTIC OVARY SYNDROME

The term 'polycystic ovary syndrome' (PCOS) covers an overlapping range of disorders which have in common:

● the presence of multiple follicular cysts in the ovaries

● inappropriate gonadotrophin secretion

● high circulating levels of androgens

● increased peripheral conversion of androgens to estrogens

● peripheral resistance to insulin.

The clinical spectrum associated with PCOS is very wide. At one extreme are asymptomatic women whose ovarian abnormality is detected biochemically or ultrasonically only. At the other extreme are women with infertility, obesity and hirsutism.

The typical polycystic ovary is enlarged and contains multiple follicular cysts (Figure 7.11) which characteristically have a prominent outer layer of luteinised thecal cells. Other features are more variable but there is commonly an increased amount of collagen in the superficial layers of the ovarian cortex, together with stromal hyperplasia and luteinisation. Numerous corpora fibrosa are usually present and corpora lutea are found in 30% of cases.

The pathophysiology of PCOS is complex. The basic abnormality appears to be an increased resistance in tissues such as fat or muscle to insulin. The ovary remains sensitive to insulin and the hyper-insulinaemia consequent to the increased peripheral insulin resistance results, via rather complex and not fully understood biochemical mechanisms, in high, non-cyclic, levels of luteinising hormone (LH), either because of an increased pituitary sensitivity to luteinising hormone-releasing hormone (LHRH) or because of increased secretion of LHRH. The high LH levels stimulate theca interna cells to produce androstenedione, which is converted in the fat cells of the body into estrone. The resulting high estrone levels then inhibit the release of follicle-stimulating hormone (FSH). Because of the low levels of FSH, follicular growth is impaired and the granulosa cells have reduced levels of aromatase and hence a decreased ability to convert androgens to estrogens. The elevated androgen levels in the ovary are thought to be responsible for the fibrous thickening of the superficial ovarian cortex, while the high circulating levels of the peripherally-produced estrone increase pituitary sensitivity to LHRH and thus perpetuate the cycle. The high estrone levels are also responsible for the development, in a proportion of these patients, of endometrial hyperplasia of simple, complex or atypical type, which may progress to an endometrial adenocarcinoma.

Ovarian malfunction is not, however, the only factor in the hormonal disturbance of PCOS. In some women, there is also an excess production of androstenedione by the adrenals.

Stromal hyperplasia and hyperthecosis

Stromal hyperplasia is characterised by varying degrees of non-neoplastic proliferation of ovarian stromal cells. Frequently associated with this is stromal hyperthecosis, in which there is focal luteinisation of the stromal cells (Figure 7.12).

Stromal hyperplasia results in a varying degree of diffuse or nodular ovarian enlargement. It occurs most commonly in the immediately postmenopausal years and is frequently asymptomatic. Some women, particularly those with associated hyperthecosis, show evidence of mild virilisation, or, less commonly, there may by hyperestrogenism because of peripheral conversion of androgens to estrone. For this reason, there is an association between stromal hyperplasia and some cases of endometrial adenocarcinoma.

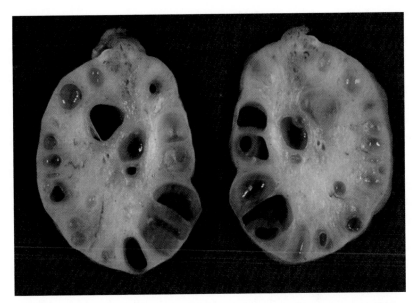

Figure 7.11. Polycystic ovary: the ovarian cortex contains numerous, thin-walled follicular cysts (reproduced with permission from Fox and Buckley, *Pathology for Gynaecologists*, 2nd ed., published by Edward Arnold)

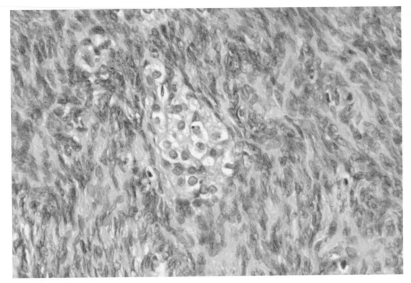

Figure 7.12. Hyperthecosis of the ovary: within the spindle-celled stroma there is a cluster of larger, luteinised cells with round nuclei and pale cytoplasm

Massive oedema of the ovary

The term 'massive oedema of the ovary' refers to a tumour-like enlargement of one or both ovaries as a result of accumulation of oedema fluid within the ovarian stroma. Massive oedema of the ovary, although quite rare, is an important and well-recognised lesion. Particularly important is its potential to present as an acute abdomen. Affected ovaries may measure up to 25 cm in diameter and, when cut, exude watery fluid. Histologically, the oedema is diffuse but usually spares the superficial cortex.

Women with massive oedema of the ovary are usually young and present with abdominal or pelvic pain, menstrual irregularities or abdominal distension. Some women are mildly virilised owing to the presence of luteinised stromal cells within the oedematous ovary.

Massive oedema of the ovary is thought to result from intermittent torsion of the ovary on its pedicle with partial obstruction of venous and lymphatic drainage. In some cases, the torsion appears to be secondary to fibromatosis of the ovary.

Luteoma of pregnancy

Luteomas of pregnancy are non-neoplastic, tumour-like, solid, yellow-brown lesions of the ovary which develop from either luteinised follicular thecal cells or from luteinised non-follicular stromal cells (Figure 7.13). The luteomas may be multiple and bilateral and may be of microscopic size only or reach up to 20 cm in diameter. Most pregnancy luteomas are discovered incidentally at caesarean section but a few are androgenic and associated with masculinisation of a female fetus or virilisation of the mother. Luteomas of pregnancy regress spontaneously during the postpartum period.

Premature ovarian failure

The term 'premature ovarian failure' is applied to those women in whom there is a cessation of ovarian function before the age of 40 years.

TRUE PREMATURE MENOPAUSE

Women with true premature menopause have high gonadotrophin levels and small ovaries in which there is a complete absence of primordial or developing follicles, although stigmata of prior ovulation are present. This condition is thought to be caused by a primary paucity

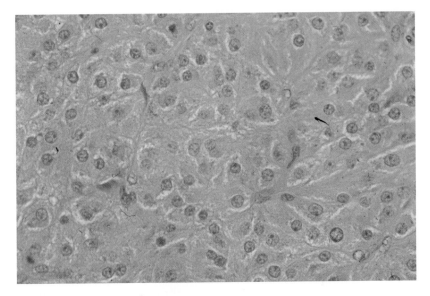

Figure 7.13. Luteoma of pregnancy

of germ cells, possibly because of inadequate migration of germ cells into the developing gonad during embryogenesis. A few cases are secondary to the use of cytotoxic drugs or radiotherapy, both of which can cause destruction of germ cells.

GONADOTROPHIN-RESISTANT OVARY SYNDROME

Gonadotrophin-resistant ovary syndrome may be congenital or acquired and is characterised by anovulation, low estrogen values and high levels of gonadotrophins. The ovary contains numerous primordial follicles, sometimes showing degenerative changes but with no evidence of follicular ripening (Figure 7.14). There is no ovarian response to the administration of exogenous gonadotrophins, even in massive doses. The syndrome has been variously attributed to a deficiency of ovarian gonadotrophin receptors, the presence of anti-gonadotrophin receptor antibodies or to a post-receptor defect.

AUTOIMMUNE OOPHORITIS

Antibodies directed against ovarian steroid-synthesising cells are found in a proportion of women with autoimmune Addison's disease. These

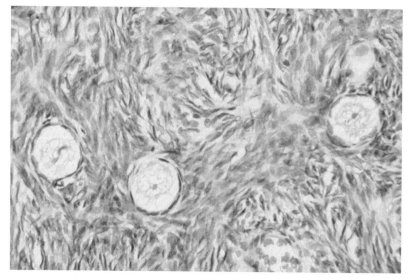

Figure 7.14. Gonadotrophin-resistant ovary: the ovarian cortex contains primordial and primary follicles but there is no evidence of follicular maturation

antibodies crossreact with steroid-synthesising cells in the adrenal glands. Women with such antibodies present with anovulatory infertility and histologically there is a lymphocytic infiltrate around secondary or tertiary follicles (Figure 7.15).

Ovarian haemorrhage

Rupture of a corpus luteum or a corpus luteum cyst may occasionally result in bleeding into the peritoneal cavity (Figure 7.16). This occurs particularly in women receiving anticoagulant therapy.

Luteinised unruptured follicle syndrome

In luteinised unruptured follicle syndrome, the follicle ripens normally but fails to release the ovum. Luteinisation of the granulosa and theca layers proceeds normally and an ovum-containing corpus luteum is formed. Hormonal activity within the ovary appears to be undisturbed, as secretory changes occur in the endometrium and thus there appears to be a primary defect in the ovum-releasing mechanism. This syndrome can be suspected if normal endometrial cyclical activity is not accompanied by ultrasonic evidence of ovulation or stigmata of ovulation on laparoscopic examination of the ovarian surface.

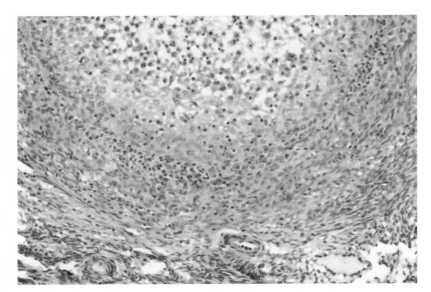

Figure 7.15. Autoimmune oophoritis: the tertiary follicle contains macrophages and lymphocytes and the wall is infiltrated by lymphocytes and occasional eosinophils: there is no ovum

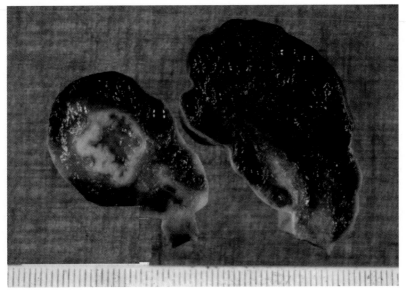

Figure 7.16. Perifollicular haematoma of the ovary: in the centre of the haematoma, the corpus luteum can be seen; intraperitoneal bleeding from such a haematoma can result in peritoneal irritation

Tumours of the ovary

There is a huge range and variety of ovarian tumours. A simplified classification of these neoplasms defines six main groups:

1 epithelial tumours

2 sex cord stromal tumours

3 germ cell tumours

4 tumours of the non-specialised tissues of the ovary

5 miscellaneous unclassified tumours

6 metastatic tumours.

EPITHELIAL TUMOURS

Epithelial tumours are neoplasms that constitute 60% of all primary ovarian tumours and 90% of those that are malignant. Most are thought to originate from undifferentiated cells in the surface or serosal epithelium of the ovary. This either arises directly from that epithelium or from epithelial fragments which have become sequestrated into the ovarian cortex to form 'epithelial inclusion cysts'. The ovarian serosa is the direct descendant and adult equivalent of the coelomic epithelium which, during embryonic life, overlies the nephrogenital ridge and from which are derived the müllerian ducts and the structures to which they give rise, namely the endocervical, endometrial and tubal epithelia. It is believed that undifferentiated cells in the ovarian surface epithelium retain a latent competence to differentiate along the same pathways as do their embryonic predecessors and that a neoplasm derived from these cells can, therefore, differentiate along various müllerian pathways. Thus, those epithelial tumours differentiating along a tubal pathway constitute the serous group of neoplasms, those differentiating along endocervical lines form the mucinous tumours, and others, which pursue an endometrial course, are classed as endometrioid tumours.

The Brenner tumour also usually develops from the ovarian serosa but this type of neoplasm is formed of uroepithelium, identical in all respects to that found in the urinary tract. Tumours of this type are therefore differentiating along wolffian rather than müllerian lines and it is not surprising that cells tracing their origin back to the coelomic epithelium of the nephrogenital ridge retain a residual capacity for differentiation along this line.

The final member of the group of epithelial ovarian neoplasms is the clear-cell tumour. This is identical in appearance to the clear-cell vaginal tumours that occur in DES-exposed girls and is certainly of a müllerian nature, although admittedly not bearing a resemblance to any adult tissue of müllerian origin. The epithelial tumours of the ovary appear to have in common, therefore, a derivation from the ovarian serosa. This unitary concept is, however, too all-embracing, for a minority of epithelial ovarian neoplasms appear to have a quite different histogenesis. Thus, some mucinous tumours are formed not of endocervical-type epithelium but of gastrointestinal-type epithelium. Most such neoplasms probably arise from areas of gastrointestinal metaplasia within the ovarian surface epithelium but some appear to be monophyletic teratomas. Furthermore, a proportion of both endometrioid and clear-cell neoplasms originate from pre-existing foci of ovarian endometriosis, while some Brenner tumours develop in the hilum of the ovary, possibly being derived from structures of wolffian origin, such as the epoophoron or epigenital tubules.

Despite these exceptions, the vast majority of epithelial neoplasms are derived from the surface epithelium and each type can exist in a benign or malignant form, the various malignant tumours sharing many common characteristics and often being considered collectively as 'ovarian adenocarcinoma'. In addition to the benign and malignant types of each neoplasm, there exists a third form, the borderline tumour (also known as 'tumour of low malignant potential' and as 'proliferating tumour').

Serous tumours

Most benign serous neoplasms are cystic, taking the form of either a simple or papillary serous cystadenoma. Serous cystadenomas are thin-walled, usually unilocular, smooth-walled cysts, measuring 3–30 cm in diameter and containing clear, straw-coloured fluid. In the papillary form of this tumour, papillae are present on one or both surfaces of the cyst. These may be few, sessile and small or numerous, large, fleshy and pedunculated (Figure 7.17). Solid, serous tumours are less common and occur either as surface serous papillomas, in which finger-like papillae project from the surface of the ovary or as serous adenofibromas, which form hard, knobbly, solid masses. Serous cystadenomas are usually lined by a single layer of flattened or cuboidal cells but in a few instances the tubal nature of the lining epithelium may be more apparent (Figure 7.18). Certainly, the true nature of the epithelium is usually more overt in the papillary neoplasms, where the central core of the papillae, formed of loose fibrous tissue, is covered by an epithelium remarkably similar to that of the fallopian tube, with secretory, ciliated and peg cells. The serous cystadenofibroma is a

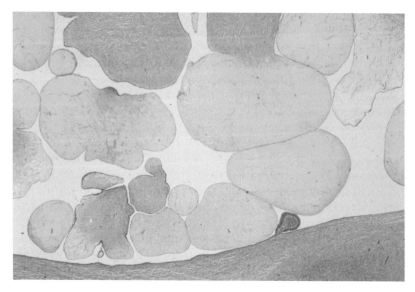

Figure 7.17. Serous papillary cystadenoma of the ovary: arising from the cyst wall (below) are oedematous, coarse papillae covered by a single layer of flattened serous epithelium

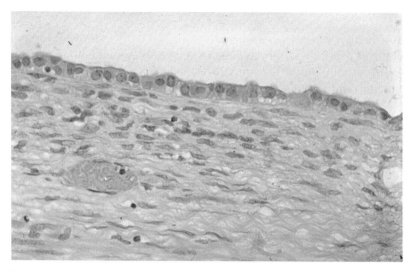

Figure 7.18. Serous cystadenoma of the ovary: the cyst is lined by a single layer of epithelium of tubal type; note the ciliated cells

predominantly fibrous tumour containing small cysts, gland-like spaces or slits lined by tubal-type epithelium.

Serous adenocarcinomas are usually large and are essentially a malignant form of the papillary serous cystadenoma, most being partially cystic and partially solid. The solid areas are formed of closely packed or merged papillae, which often penetrate through the outer capsule of the neoplasm. Foci of necrosis or haemorrhage are common and any fluid present in the cystic portion of the tumour is commonly blood stained. Histologically, well-differentiated serous adenocarcinomas retain a papillary pattern but the epithelium shows multilayering, irregular tufting, nuclear hyperchromatism, pleomorphism and mitotic activity, whilst stromal invasion is readily apparent (Figure 7.19). From this clearly papillary form, there is a spectrum of differentiation extending through to the diffuse pattern in which the tumour grows in solid sheets of cells.

Mucinous tumours

Benign mucinous tumours are almost invariably cystic, taking the form of a mucinous cystadenoma. These cystic neoplasms commonly measure 15–30 cm in diameter but can attain a huge size and fill the abdominal cavity. The cysts have a thick, parchment-like wall and are usually multilocular, the locules characteristically containing clear, tenacious mucoid material. Histologically, the walls of the locules are formed of fibrous tissue and the cyst is lined by a single layer of tall, mucus-containing cells (Figure 7.20). In most tumours, the epithelium is identical to that of the endocervix, but in a proportion the epithelium is of enteric type, containing goblet cells, argyrophil cells and occasionally Paneth cells.

Mucinous adenocarcinomas are usually either partially or wholly solid. Areas of necrosis or haemorrhage are common and mucoid material often exudes from their cut surface. These neoplasms show a wide spectrum of differentiation, ranging from a well-marked acinar or glandular pattern (Figure 7.21) to one in which the tumour is formed largely of solid sheets of cells in which intracellular mucus is usually present.

Mucinous tumours of any type, but usually in the benign or borderline categories, may be complicated by pseudomyxoma peritonei in which there is a marked accumulation of mucoid material in the peritoneal cavity. This has traditionally been attributed to leakage from the ovarian tumour but it has become apparent that in most, possibly all, cases there is an associated neoplasm of the appendix or, less commonly, the intestine. It has been suggested that the pseudomyxoma peritonei is

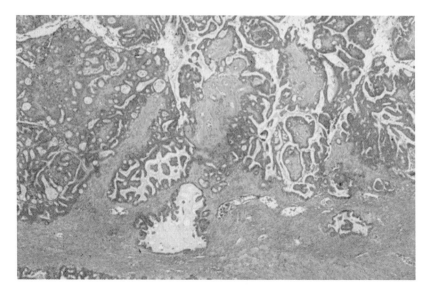

Figure 7.19. Well-differentiated serous adenocarcinoma of the ovary: the tumour is composed of fibrous papillae covered by epithelium in which there is extensive budding and proliferation

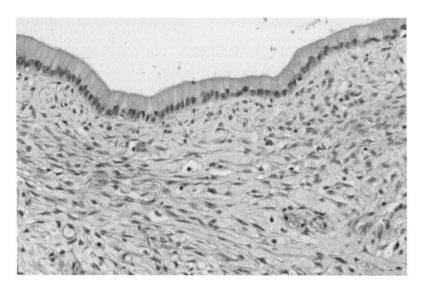

Figure 7.20. Mucinous cyst of the ovary: the cyst is lined by a single layer of tall columnar, mucin-secreting epithelium: the cells are similar to those seen in the endocervix

secondary to the gastrointestinal lesion and that the apparently primary ovarian tumours in such cases are, despite their non-malignant appearance, metastases from the appendicular or intestinal neoplasm.

Endometrioid tumours

Benign endometrioid tumours appear to be very rare, although occasional examples of an endometrioid adenoma or adenofibroma are encountered. The former tends to resemble an endometrial polyp while the latter is a neoplasm resembling the serous adenofibroma but in which the enclosed glands are lined by an endometrial-type epithelium. This apparent paucity of benign endometrioid tumours may, however, be more apparent than real, as it is probable that many of the lesions classed as endometriotic cysts of the ovary are, in reality, benign endometrioid cystadenomas.

Endometrioid adenocarcinomas may be solid, partially cystic or wholly cystic, the latter variety usually showing abundant papillary in-growths. The defining histological feature of an endometrioid adeno-carcinoma is that it mimics exactly an endometrial adenocarcinoma (Figure 7.22). Most are well differentiated and have an acinar pattern but in a minority there is a predominantly sheet-like pattern of growth. It is worth noting that any neoplasm which occurs in the endometrium can also arise in the ovary as a variant of an adenocarcinoma and thus carcinosarcomas, adenosarcomas and stromal sarcomas can all occur in the ovary as forms of endometrioid neoplasia.

Brenner tumours

The majority of Brenner tumours are benign and occur as small, solid, well-circumscribed nodules with a smooth or bosselated surface and a hard, whorled, greyish-white, cut surface. Histologically, the Brenner tumour is characterised by well-demarcated nests and branching columns of epithelial cells set in a fibrous stroma (Figure 7.23). The epithelial nests are formed of round or polygonal cells with distinct limiting membranes, abundant cytoplasm and ovoid or round nuclei, which are often prominently grooved. Cystic change in the centre of the cell nests is common and these cystic spaces may be lined by flattened, cuboidal or columnar cells.

Malignant Brenner tumours may resemble architecturally a benign Brenner neoplasm but show a marked overgrowth of the epithelial component with nuclear hyperchromatism, cytological atypia, mitotic activity and stromal invasion. Some malignant Brenner tumours develop as pure transitional cell carcinomas (Figure 7.24). Such tumours are, however, controversial because, despite their morphological resemblance

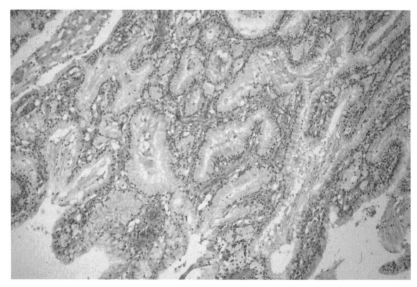

Figure 7.21. Well-differentiated mucinous adenocarcinoma of the ovary: the neoplasm consists of glandular acini lined by a mucus-secreting epithelium

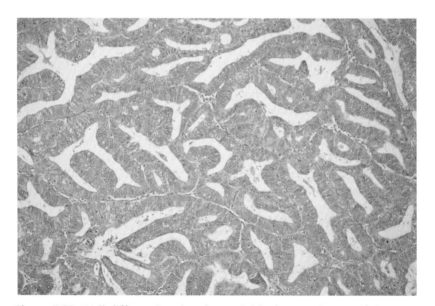

Figure 7.22. Well-differentiated endometrioid adenocarcinoma of the ovary: the tumour is similar in appearance to an adenocarcinoma of the endometrium

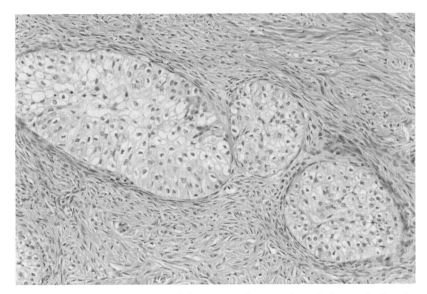

Figure 7.23. Brenner tumour of the ovary: the neoplasm is formed of well-demarcated nests of transitional epithelium set in a fibrous stroma

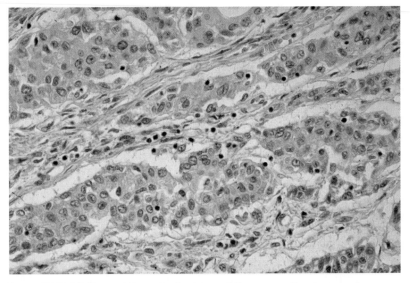

Figure 7.24. Malignant Brenner tumour of the ovary: the tumour is composed of highly atypical, infiltrating transitional epithelium

to urothelium, they do not exhibit the immunohistochemical profile of urothelium.

Clear-cell tumours

Benign clear-cell neoplasms are distinctly uncommon and take the form of clear-cell adenofibromas in which gland-like spaces set in fibrous tissue are lined by cells with clear cytoplasm and hobnail nuclei. Most clear-cell tumours are adenocarcinomas. These are usually large and only a minority are solid, most being cystic with solid areas. The solid areas tend to be soft and fleshy, whereas the cystic portions are commonly multilocular and often contain mucoid material. These neoplasms have a complex histological appearance, showing an admixture of papillary, cystic, glandular and solid growth forms (Figure 7.25). The cysts and acini tend to be lined by cells with clear cytoplasm and large, deeply-staining nuclei which protrude into the lumen (hobnail nuclei).

Ovarian adenocarcinoma

The malignant forms of the various epithelial tumours of the ovary are, in clinical practice, commonly grouped together into the single entity of ovarian adenocarcinoma. Serous and endometrioid tumours form the bulk of ovarian adenocarcinoma. Mucinous tumours are less common and clear-cell carcinoma and malignant Brenner tumours are relatively rare. It has been widely believed that tumour type is of some prognostic significance with, for example, serous adenocarcinomas pursuing a more malignant course than do their endometrioid counterparts. Multivariate analysis has, however, shown that this is generally not the case, although late stage mucinous and possibly clear-cell adenocarcinomas do have an unduly poor prognosis because of their resistance to platinum-based chemotherapy. In the case of mucinous tumours, this may be due to the fact that some of them are actually of gastrointestinal, rather than ovarian, origin. The two most significant prognostic factors are the clinical stage at the time of diagnosis and the histological grade of the neoplasm.

Staging of ovarian adenocarcinomas is dependent upon a knowledge of their mode of spread. Local spread is by direct seeding on to the peritoneum, with implantation of secondary deposits in the contralateral ovary, the pouch of Douglas, the omentum and the surface of the uterus. Malignant cells are also seeded into the small amount of fluid that is normally present in the peritoneal cavity. This fluid tends to circulate upwards along the paracolic gutters and, whereas on the left side the circulation of the fluid is dammed by the

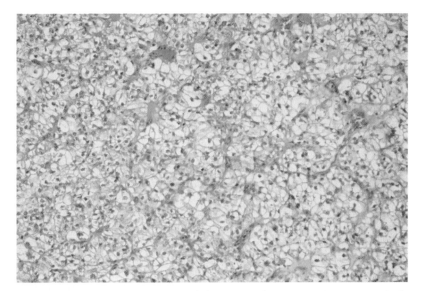

Figure 7.25. Clear-cell carcinoma of the ovary: the tumour is composed of sheets of cells with clear cytoplasm

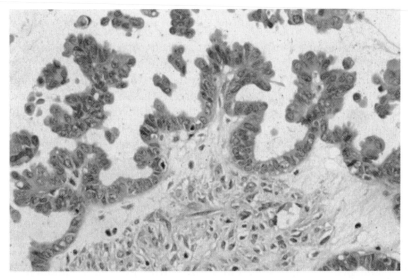

Figure 7.26. A borderline serous tumour: the cells covering the papillae are multilayered, rather pleomorphic and show irregular budding; there is no stromal invasion

phrenicocolic ligament, there is no such bar on the right side of the abdomen and the fluid reaches the under surface of the right leaf of the diaphragm. Tumour cells are thus carried into the paracolic gutters and to the right leaf of the diaphragm, these being sites of early metastasis. Lymphatic spread is to the pelvic nodes. Spread to the para-aortic nodes also occurs, at a relatively early stage in the growth of the tumour. Blood-borne spread is a late and uncommon event and is usually to the liver and lungs.

Currently, ovarian adenocarcinoma has a gloomy prognosis, the overall 5-year survival rate being only in the region of 25–30%. Unfortunately, little is known of the aetiology of this lethal form of neoplasia. It has been suggested that the ground is prepared for eventual neoplastic change in the surface epithelium by the repetitive minor trauma of ovulation, a view lent credence by the finding that both oral contraception and pregnancy, each associated with inhibition of ovulation, decrease the risk of developing ovarian adenocarcinoma. The protective effect of pregnancy is cumulative but, nevertheless, simple inhibition of ovulation is not the entire explanation for these effects, for one pregnancy offers the same degree of protection as does 3 years' use of oral contraceptives.

Genetic factors are also important and about 5% of ovarian cancers develop in women with mutations of 'ovarian cancer genes' such as the *BRCA1* and *BRCA2* genes; such tumours are usually of serous type.

Borderline epithelial tumours

Borderline epithelial tumours are neoplasms that are also known as 'tumours of low malignant potential' or 'proliferative tumours'. They lie in the grey area between clearly benign and overtly malignant epithelial ovarian neoplasms. It is largely the serous and mucinous borderline tumours which have been defined, with borderline endometrioid, Brenner and clear-cell neoplasms being less well delineated. The borderline serous neoplasms have been a subject of dispute in recent years. Some have denied their existence and have maintained that tumours classed as being of borderline malignancy are, in reality, low-grade adenocarcinomas. Similar doubts have also been expressed about borderline mucinous neoplasms but never the less it is widely thought that borderline serous and mucinous tumours should be retained as distinct entities. They are relatively common and macroscopically closely resemble their fully benign counterparts.

Histologically (Figures 7.26 and 7.27), the epithelial component of these neoplasms shows some or indeed all of the characteristics of malignancy, such as multilayering, irregular budding, cytological

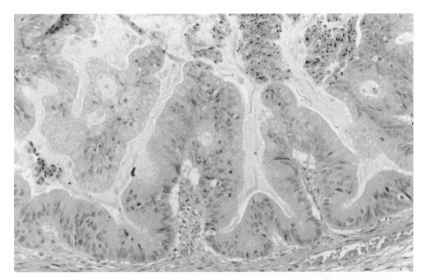

Figure 7.27. A borderline mucinous tumour of intestinal type: the locule is lined by columnar, mucin-secreting cells in which there is loss of nuclear polarity, nuclear pleomorphism and which form tufts and irregular papillae

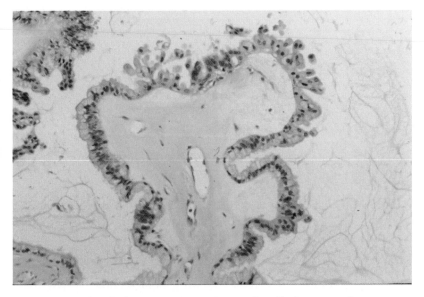

Figure 7.28. A borderline mucinous tumour of müllerian type: the tumour locules are lined by coarse papillae covered by mucinous cells of endocervical type in which there is irregular budding and nuclear pleomorphism

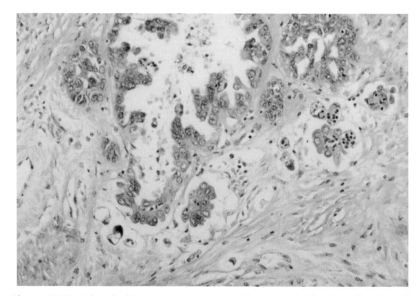

Figure 7.29. A borderline serous tumour with stromal microinvasion. Small clusters of atypical serous cells arise from the cyst lining and penetrate the surrounding stroma

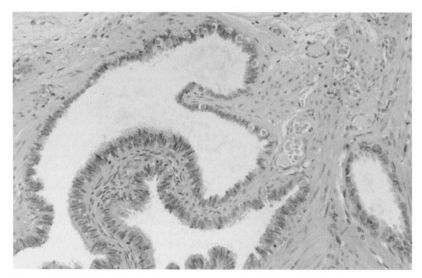

Figure 7.30. Endosalpingiosis: a cluster of glands lined by benign serous epithelium lies in the subperitoneal stroma (reproduced with permission from Fox and Buckley, *Atlas of Gynaecological Pathology*, published by MTP Press

atypia, nuclear hyperchromatism and pleomorphism and mitotic activity. There is, however, no stromal invasion and this lack of invasiveness is both a defining feature of these neoplasms and an indication of their unique biological status. The tumours, particularly those of serous type, may show a homogeneously borderline pattern throughout, or there may be an admixture, within a single neoplasm, of clearly benign epithelium and of epithelium showing borderline characteristics. It must be stressed that the diagnosis of a tumour of borderline malignancy is a positive one that is based on the histological findings and that the use of this term is not indicative of any indecision on the pathologist's part as to whether the tumour is benign or malignant.

Mucinous tumours of borderline malignancy form two distinct groups: those in which the epithelium is of intestinal type (Figure 7.27) and those in which the epithelium is of müllerian or endocervical type (Figure 7.28). The latter resemble the serous tumours in that they tend to form papillary cystic neoplasms unlike the intestinal type which tend to have smooth cystic linings.

In a small proportion of serous and mucinous tumours of borderline malignancy, there may be microscopic foci of invasion limited to the neoplastic stroma (Figure 7.29). The clinical significance of this finding is currently the subject of debate.

In a proportion of borderline tumours, particularly and perhaps only those of serous type, there appears to be extraovarian spread with multiple small tumour nodules dotted around on the peritoneum and omentum. Some of these are possibly seedling implants from neoplasms with an exophytic growth pattern but most are not true metastases, developing in situ within the submesothelial connective tissues (the secondary müllerian system). Histologically, these may show a fully benign pattern (endosalpingiosis, Figure 7.30), a pattern resembling that seen in a borderline tumour (atypical endosalpingiosis) or desmoplastic peritoneal implants (Figure 7.31) or can appear invasive and resemble true metastases from an adenocarcinoma. The latter is entirely consistent with a diagnosis of borderline serous tumour based on the histological findings in the primary ovarian neoplasm. It is important for prognosis for primary peritoneal serous carcinoma associated with an ovarian tumour of borderline malignancy to be distinguished from implants of borderline tumour, as the former has a poorer outcome. If peritoneal lesions do progress, they do so in an indolent fashion. Tumours of borderline malignancy without extra-ovarian lesions have an excellent prognosis. A micropapillary pattern of serous borderline tumour is more likely to be associated with invasive peritoneal disease.

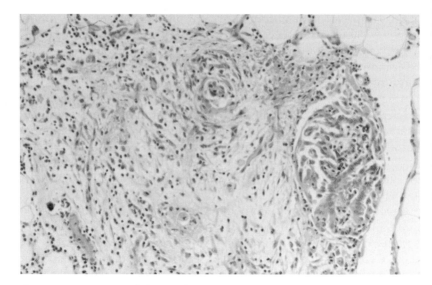

Figure 7.31. Peritoneal desmoplastic serous implant: this is an implant into the peritoneum of fragments of borderline serous tumour; the papillary nature of the implant (to the right) and the fibrous and inflammatory response to the implant can be seen

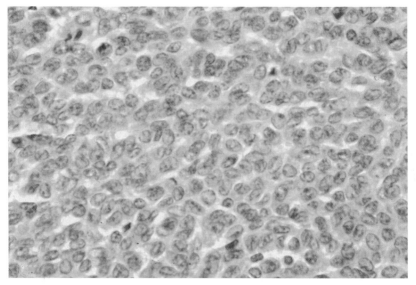

Figure 7.32. Adult type granulosa cell tumour of the ovary, diffuse pattern: the solid tumour is composed of uniform oval cells with evenly stained and grooved nuclei

SEX CORD STROMAL TUMOURS

The neoplasms contain granulosa cells, Sertoli cells, thecal cells, Leydig cells, fibroblasts of specialised stromal origin or the precursors of these cells, either singly or in any combination. It has been thought that all these cells are ultimately derived from the mesenchyme of the genital ridge but it is more likely that both granulosa and Sertoli cells differentiate from the sex cords of the developing gonad. These cords probably originate from the coelomic epithelium rather than from mesenchyme. It is believed that sex cord cells can, depending on the nature of the developing gonad, differentiate into either Sertoli or granulosa cells, and that this bisexual potentiality is retained in undifferentiated sex cord cells in the adult gonad; granulosa cell tumours and Sertoli cell neoplasms thus being homologous with each other. Neoplasia of these cells is often accompanied by a reactive stromal proliferation which, in the case of a granulosa cell tumour, often shows thecomatous differentiation and in Sertoli cell neoplasms shows Leydig cell differentiation. Pure stromal neoplasms, thecomas and Leydig cell tumours can also occur.

Granulosa cell tumours, adult type

Adult type granulosa cell tumours are usually solid neoplasms which may be hard or rubbery. Their cut surface is white, yellow or grey and their average size is about 12 cm in diameter. A proportion of granulosa cell neoplasms are, however, partially cystic and a few are wholly cystic, resembling a cystadenoma.

Histologically, the cells in a granulosa cell tumour are small, round or polygonal, having little cytoplasm and indistinct cell boundaries (Figure 7.32). Their large, round or ovoid pale nuclei characteristically show longitudinal grooving. The cells are arranged in a variety of patterns and, although in any individual neoplasm a particular pattern may predominate, there is usually an admixture of cellular arrangements. In the insular pattern, the cells are arranged in compact masses or islands, whereas in the trabecular pattern the cells form anastomosing ribbons or cords (Figure 7.33). Alternatively, the cells may be arranged in sheets to give a diffuse pattern (Figure 7.32). In the microfollicular pattern, granulosa cells are arranged around small spaces containing nuclear fragments, these being the Call–Exner bodies (Figure 7.34), while a macrofollicular pattern is caused by liquefaction within islands of granulosa cells. In cystic granulosa cell tumours, the cyst lining resembles that of a graafian follicle but usually contains microfollicles.

A granulosa cell tumour may produce non-specific pelvic tumour

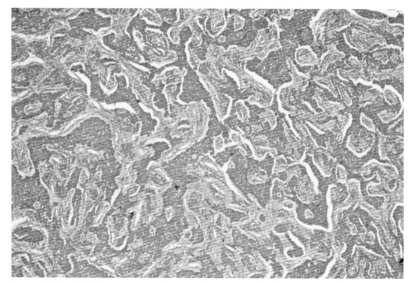

Figure 7.33. Adult type granulosa cell tumour of the ovary with a trabecular pattern: the tumour cells form anastomosing cords and ribbons (reproduced with permission from Fox and Buckley, *Atlas of Gynaecological Pathology*, published by MTP Press)

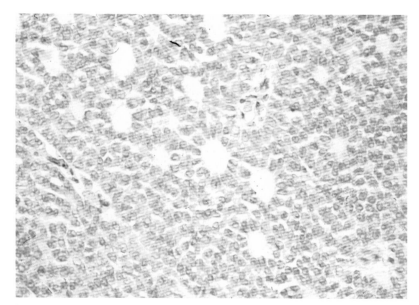

Figure 7.34. Adult type granulosa cell tumour of the ovary with a microfollicular pattern. Call–Exner bodies are present

symptoms but about 75% of women with such neoplasms have symptoms indicative of estrogen secretion by the neoplasm. Thus, in young girls these tumours commonly result in isosexual precocious pseudopuberty, whereas in women of reproductive age complaints of irregular menstruation or menorrhagia are common. In post-menopausal women, granulosa cell tumours cause postmenopausal vaginal bleeding and sometimes a resurgence of libido. Endometrial changes, such as simple or atypical hyperplasia, are commonly found in association with granulosa cell tumours, while an endometrial adenocarcinoma occurs in 6–10% of cases. A few granulosa cell tumours, particularly those which are cystic, appear to be androgenic rather than estrogenic.

All granulosa cell tumours should be considered as potentially malignant, although the degree of malignancy is often very low and the course pursued by the tumour is frequently very indolent. Recurrence or metastases tend to occur late, commonly after 5 years, not infrequently after 10 years and sometimes after 20 years. The histological pattern of the tumour is of no prognostic importance; indeed it is doubtful if there are any prognostic indicators apart from extraovarian spread. The long-term survival rate for women with this neoplasm is between 50% and 60%. Inhibin may be used both as an immunohistochemical and serum marker of granulosa cell tumours, reflecting its physiological production by normal granulosa cells.

Juvenile granulosa cell tumour

Juvenile granulosa cell tumour is a histological variant of granulosa cell tumour which occurs predominantly in women aged less than 20 years, although some neoplasms of this type arise in older women. The tumours (Figure 7.35) contain follicles and cysts lined by granulosa cells, together with solid areas showing a haphazard admixture of granulosa and thecal cells, which can show a striking degree of luteinisation. The neoplastic cells lack the nuclear grooving characteristic of an adult-type granulosa cell tumour and there is often a moderate degree of cytological atypia and mitotic activity.

About 5% of juvenile granulosa cell tumours behave in a malignant fashion and tend to recur rapidly and disseminate widely throughout the abdominal cavity within 2 years of the initial diagnosis, a pattern of malignant behaviour quite unlike that of an adult-type granulosa cell tumour.

Thecomas (fibrothecoma)

Thecomas are solid tumours (Figure 7.36) formed of plump, pale, ovoid

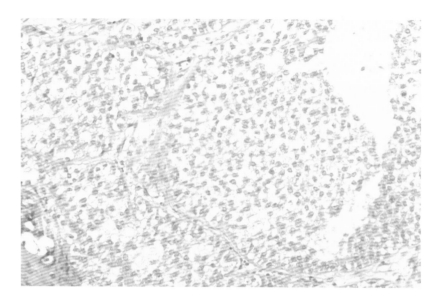

Figure 7.35. Juvenile granulosa cell tumour of the ovary: regular pale-staining granulosa cells line the wall of a macrofollicle

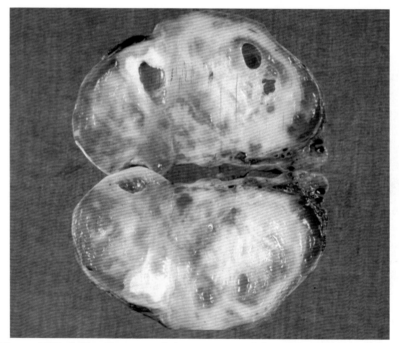

Figure 7.36. A fibrothecoma of the ovary: a mainly solid neoplasm with some small areas of cystic degeneration

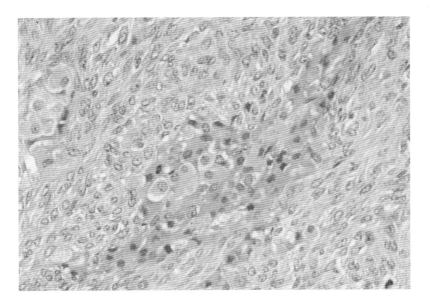

Figure 7.37. A thecoma of the ovary: the tumour cells are oval to round with indistinct borders and the cells in the centre of the field have eosinophilic cytoplasm indicative of luteinisation

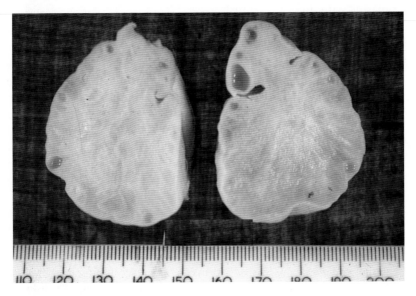

Figure 7.38. A fibroma of the ovary: a firm, predominantly solid neoplasm with small areas of cystic degeneration

or spindle-shaped cells with indistinct borders arranged in interlacing bundles or anastomosing trabeculae. These neoplasms arise from the ovarian mesenchyme and occur most commonly in postmenopausal women. They are estrogenic and produce symptoms similar to those noted in patients with granulosa cell tumours. Some thecomas show focal luteinisation and such neoplasms may be weakly androgenic (Figure 7.37). Thecomas are, with rare exceptions, benign. Malignant thecomas are not distinguishable from fibrosarcomas.

Fibromas

Neoplasms of the fibroma type probably arise from ovarian gonadal stroma (Figure 7.38). They are similar to fibromas elsewhere in the body but it is of note that a proportion of ovarian fibromas are, for unknown reasons, accompanied by ascites and a hydrothorax (Meig's syndrome). Ovarian fibromas also tend to occur in association with the basal cell naevus or Gorlin's syndrome, under which unusual circumstances the tumours tend to be bilateral, multifocal and calcified. Fibromas are benign but a few show increased cellularity (Figure 7.39), pleomorphism and mitotic activity. Tumours showing these features to only a mild degree are classed as cellular fibromas which will recur if incompletely removed. Those with more marked atypia and mitotic activity are classed as fibrosarcomas. These are highly aggressive neoplasms with a poor prognosis.

Androblastoma

Androblastomas are neoplasms composed of Sertoli cells, Leydig cells or a combination of the two cell types. Pure Sertoli cell neoplasms are rare and occur as small, solid, yellowish masses. Histologically (Figure 7.40), the tumours show highly differentiated tubules lined by a single layer of radially orientated Sertoli cells which commonly contain lipid droplets and are occasionally distended and vacuolated by fat. Sertoli cell neoplasms are, with very rare exceptions, benign and about 50% appear to be estrogenic, the remainder lacking any obvious endocrinological activity.

Leydig cell neoplasms may arise either from stromal cells or from pre-existing hilar cells. The tumours are small, yellowish-brown and consist of Leydig cells arranged in sheets or solid cords (Figure 7.41). The cytoplasm of the Leydig cells is markedly eosinophilic and their nuclei are large and centrally placed. Reinke's crystals, slender rod-shaped bodies with rounded, tapering or square ends, are present in the cytoplasm of about 50% of these neoplasms but are irregularly distributed and often difficult to detect.

Leydig cell tumours are nearly always virilising, although occasional estrogenic or endocrinologically inert examples are encountered. The vast majority (95%) are benign but exceptional tumours of this type give rise to metastases, a possibility not predictable on any histological grounds.

Sertoli–Leydig cell tumours are generally solid neoplasms showing a wide range of histological differentiation. Well-differentiated neoplasms are formed of tubules lined by Sertoli cells with variable numbers of Leydig cells between the tubules. In less well-differentiated tumours, the Sertoli cells are arranged in cords, solid tubules or trabeculae (Figure 7.42), these being set in a mesenchymal stroma containing clusters or nodules of Leydig cells. Poorly differentiated Sertoli–Leydig neoplasms (Figure 7.43) consist largely of sheets of spindle-shaped cells in which occasional irregular cord-like structures or imperfectly formed tubules may be recognised with Leydig cells also present in small clusters.

Sertoli–Leydig cell neoplasms can occur at any age but the majority develop in women aged between 10 and 35 years. These tumours are usually androgenic and produce virilisation. The well-differentiated neoplasms always behave in a benign fashion but between 10% and 40% of the less well-differentiated tumours behave in a malignant fashion, this being particularly the case for the poorly-differentiated tumours.

Recurrence or metastases, characteristically to the omentum, abdominal lymph nodes or liver, are usually apparent within one year of initial diagnosis.

Gynandroblastoma

A true gynandroblastoma contains an admixture of areas showing unequivocal granulosa cell differentiation and of other areas in which there is equally incontrovertible Sertoli cell differentiation. Such tumours are extremely rare and, consequently, their pattern of behaviour is still largely undetermined.

Sex cord tumour with annular tubules

This uncommon but histologically distinctive sex cord tumour contains rounded nests in which epithelial-like cells surround hyaline bodies (Figure 7.44). The epithelial-like cells, which are thought to be immature sex cord cells, are palisaded along the periphery of the cell nests and around the hyaline bodies. About one-third of these tumours are associated with the Peutz–Jeghers syndrome and, in such circumstances, the lesions are usually bilateral, of microscopic size, calcified and benign. The tumours not associated with the Peutz–Jeghers

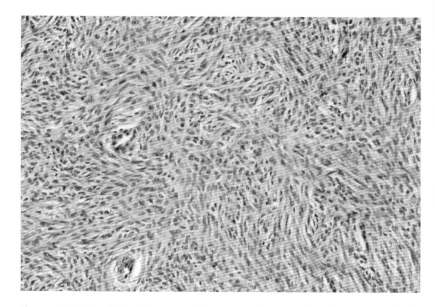

Figure 7.39. A cellular fibroma of the ovary: the neoplasm is composed of spindle cells arranged in interweaving bundles

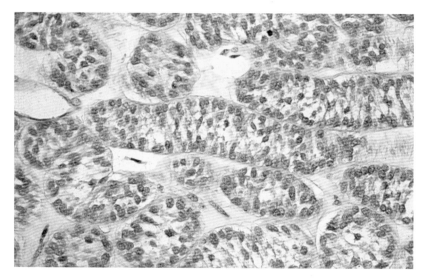

Figure 7.40. Sertoli cell tumour of the ovary: the tumour is composed, throughout, of narrow tubules lined by radially orientated Sertoli cells, set in a fibrous stroma

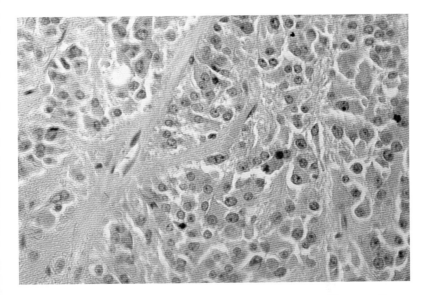

Figure 7.41. Leydig cell tumour of the ovary: the tumour cells are uniform in shape but the nuclei are grouped and irregularly dispersed

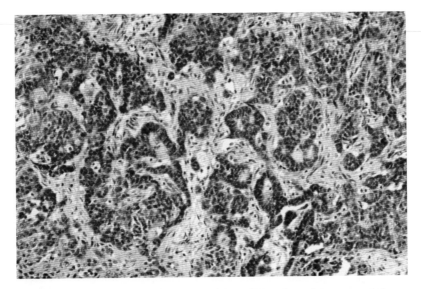

Figure 7.42. Moderately differentiated Sertoli-Leydig cell tumour of the ovary: the neoplasm is composed of darkly staining cells, resembling sex cords, set in a fibrous stroma in which there are small numbers of eosinophilic-staining Leydig cells

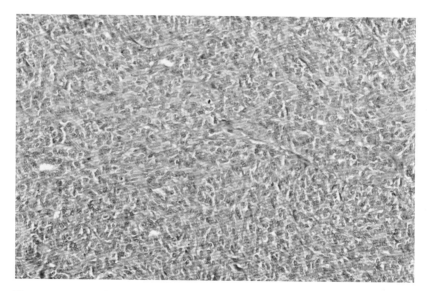

Figure 7.43. Poorly differentiated Sertoli-Leydig cell tumour of the ovary: the neoplasm is solid and composed of bundles of spindle-shaped cells admixed with small numbers of Leydig cells

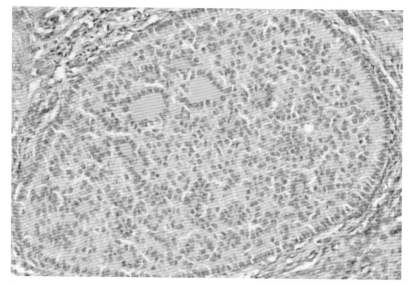

Figure 7.44. Sex cord tumour with annular tubules: the neoplasm is composed of discrete islands of immature sex cord cells palisaded around the periphery of the islands and around amorphous proteinaceous material

syndrome are unilateral, large, uncalcified, often show an overgrowth of either granulosa or Sertoli cells and behave in a malignant fashion in about 20% of cases.

GERM CELL TUMOURS

Tumours derived from germ cells may show no evidence of differentiation into either embryonic or extra-embryonic tissues. They can differentiate into embryonic tissue or may differentiate along extra-embryonic pathways into trophoblast or yolk sac structures. Very little is known about the aetiology of germ cell neoplasms. Extensive studies of naturally-occurring gonadal teratomas in highly inbred genetic strains of mice and of experimentally induced murine teratomas have, however, indicated that teratomas arise from pathogenetic pregnancies (that is, in which there has been no fertilisation of the ovum) which undergo a short period of embryogenesis and then break up to yield a neoplasm. Genetic studies of human ovarian teratomas strongly suggest that these tumours arise in a similar manner.

Dysgerminoma

Dysgerminoma is a neoplasm formed of cells which closely resemble primordial germ cells, showing no evidence of differentiation into either embryonic or extra-embryonic structures. As such, the tumour is identical to the seminoma of the testis. Dysgerminomas commonly arise in women aged between 10 and 30 years. Their development is usually announced by non-specific tumour symptoms, although isosexual precocious pseudopuberty is sometimes seen in young girls. These neoplasms have a particular tendency to arise in women with developmental abnormalities of the gonads, although the vast majority of dysgerminomas occur in otherwise fully normal individuals.

The tumours are solid and usually measure about 12 cm in diameter. Histologically (Figure 7.45), the neoplastic cells are large, uniform, round, oval or polyhedral, with well-defined limiting membranes, abundant cytoplasm and large vesicular nuclei. The cells are commonly arranged in solid nests separated by delicate fibrous septa but may form cords or strands embedded in a fibrous stroma. A lymphocytic infiltration of the stroma, sometimes aggregated into follicles with germinal centres and small stromal granulomas, are characteristic features.

Dysgerminomas are malignant. Rupture of their enveloping 'capsule' often leads to direct implantation of tumour onto the pelvic peritoneum and omentum and lymphatic spread occurs relatively early to the para-aortic, retroperitoneal, mediastinal and supraclavicular nodes. Haematogenous spread to the liver, lungs, kidneys and bone occurs at a late stage. These tumours are, however, highly sensitive to both radiation and chemotherapy and the 5-year survival rate is well over 90%.

Choriocarcinomas

Choriocarcinomas are germ cell tumours showing trophoblastic differentiation. They are often combined with other malignant germ cell elements but pure ovarian choriocarcinomas are occasionally encountered. In women of reproductive age, it is usually impossible to tell whether such a neoplasm is a germ cell tumour, a metastasis from a uterine choriocarcinoma or a tumour arising from the placental tissue of an ectopic ovarian pregnancy. In premenarchal and postmenopausal women, this problem does not arise and, here, an origin from ovarian germ cells can be readily accepted. The histological appearances of such tumours are identical to those of gestational uterine choriocarcinomas. Nevertheless, ovarian choriocarcinomas respond poorly to the chemotherapeutic regimen which is so successful for uterine gestational choriocarcinomas.

Yolk sac tumours

Yolk sac tumours are rare neoplasms, also known as endodermal sinus tumours, which represent neoplastic germ cell differentiation along extra-embryonic lines into mesoblast and yolk sac endoderm. They share with yolk sac structures the ability to secrete α-fetoprotein (AFP). Yolk sac tumours form large masses showing conspicuous haemorrhage, necrosis and microcystic change. Their histological appearances are very complex (Figure 7.46) but there is characteristically a loose vacuolated labyrinthine network containing microcysts lined by flattened cells together with Schiller–Duval bodies. These bodies have a mesenchymal core containing a central capillary and an epithelial investment of cuboidal or columnar cells. A glandular pattern is often seen and there may be hepatoid or endodermal differentiation. Eosinophilic hyaline droplets are present in nearly all yolk sac tumours and these consist predominantly of AFP.

Yolk sac tumours occur most commonly in girls aged 4–20 years. They present solely with non-specific tumour symptoms and are highly aggressive neoplasms which spread rapidly within the abdomen and to distant sites. Their previously appalling prognosis has been much improved by the introduction of effective chemotherapy and the prognosis is now relatively hopeful in a substantial proportion of cases. The progress of the tumour, its response to chemotherapy and the development of recurrence can all be monitored by serial estimations of serum AFP levels.

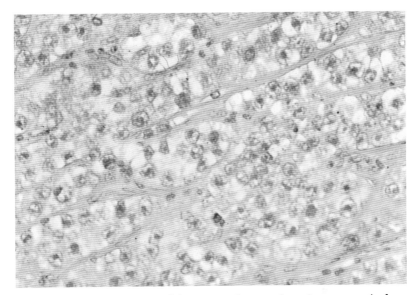

Figure 7.45. Dysgerminoma of the ovary: the neoplasm is composed of undifferentiated germ cells with vesicular nuclei and clear cytoplasm which are arranged in trabeculae

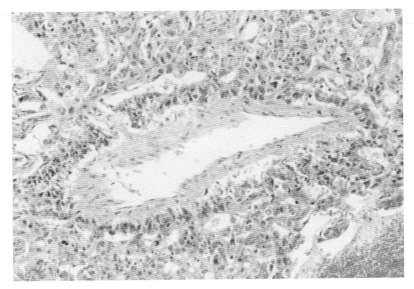

Figure 7.46. Yolk sac tumour of the ovary: in the centre of the field there is a Schiller–Duval body with a central blood vessel surrounded by tumour cells in which there is a perivascular space

Teratomas

Teratomas are germ cell neoplasms showing differentiation along embryonic lines. In most, there is a melange of tissues but in some, known as monophyletic teratomas, there is differentiation along only a single tissue pathway, for example solely into thyroid tissue. The terms 'benign' and 'malignant' are not truly applicable to teratomas, for the prognosis of any individual neoplasm is determined not by the usual criteria of malignancy but by the degree of maturity of its constituent tissues. Those in which all the components are fully mature behave in a benign fashion and increasing degrees of tissue immaturity are associated with a progressive tendency towards the neoplasm running a malignant course. Hence, teratomas are classed as either 'immature' or 'mature', the term 'malignant' being reserved for those cases in which true malignant change has occurred in a mature teratoma, such as when a squamous cell carcinoma develops in a mature cystic teratoma.

The vast majority of ovarian teratomas are mature and cystic. Such neoplasms, often known as 'dermoids', account for between 10% and 20% of all ovarian tumours and for 97% of ovarian teratomas, these being usually cystic. Just over 10% of mature cystic teratomas are bilateral. Most measure between 5 cm and 15 cm in diameter and some are pedunculated. They are round or ovoid with a smooth or slightly wrinkled outer surface. On opening, the teratomas are usually unilocular and have a smooth or granular inner surface. There is commonly a focal hillock-like protuberance into the cyst lumen, this being usually known as Rokitansky's tubercle or the mamillary body. The cysts nearly always contain greasy sebaceous material and hair. Teeth are present in about one-third and these may lie loose in the cyst; they may be embedded in the wall or attached to a rudimentary jaw bone. Histologically, the cyst is almost invariably lined by squamous epithelium and skin appendages are also common (Figure 7.47). Fat, respiratory-type epithelium, bone, cartilage, neural tissue, gastro-intestinal-type epithelium, thyroid and salivary gland tissue are frequent components. Breast or pituitary tissue is uncommonly encountered and some tissues, such as kidney, pancreas and spleen, are noticeable for their almost complete absence. There is currently no explanation for this apparent selectivity.

Ninety percent of mature cystic teratomas are found in women of reproductive age and most are asymptomatic incidental findings. However, some women suffer complications such as torsion or rupture, both of which present as an acute abdominal emergency. Sometimes a rupture is less acute and slow leakage of cyst contents produces a

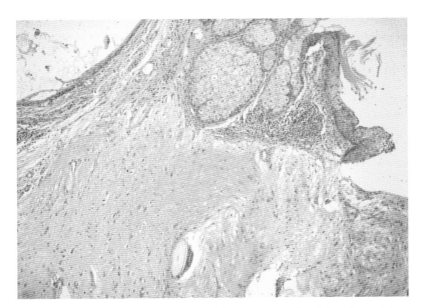

Figure 7.47. Mature cystic teratoma of the ovary: to the right, the cyst is lined by mature stratified squamous epithelium and the wall contains sebaceous glands above and neuroepithelium below, in which a hair is embedded

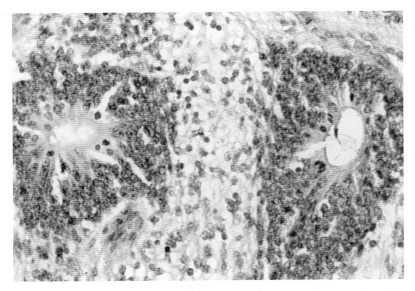

Figure 7.48. Immature teratoma of the ovary: there two clusters of rosette-like structures which are composed of immature neuroepithelium

chronic chemical peritonitis. Occasionally, women present with a haemolytic anaemia due, it is believed, to the presence of tumour antigens, which evoke antibodies that cross-react with erythrocytic antigens.

True malignant change occurs in 1–2% of women with mature cystic teratomas, this usually taking the form of a squamous cell carcinoma.

A small proportion of mature teratomas are solid rather than cystic but most solid teratomas are of the immature variety. These are rare neoplasms which occur principally during the first two decades of life. Microscopic examination of such neoplasms reveals an admixture of both mature and immature tissues, although immature mesenchyme or neuro-epithelium (Figure 7.48) tend to be dominant features. Immature teratomas behave in a malignant fashion, implanting on to pelvic peritoneum, metastasising to retroperitoneal and para-aortic lymph nodes and being disseminated via the bloodstream to the lungs and liver. The previously extremely poor prognosis of these neoplasms has been transformed by chemotherapy, with approximately 60% of patients now surviving.

Monophyletic teratomas, in which differentiation is into only one tissue, are characterised by the struma ovarii which consists solely or predominantly of tissue that is histologically, physiologically and pharmacologically identical to that of the normal thyroid gland (Figure 7.49). This ovarian thyroid tissue may function autonomously to produce a 'pelvic' hyperthyroidism; it can show the changes of a lymphocytic thyroiditis and sometimes undergoes malignant change with a resulting thyroid adenocarcinoma which can metastasise to lymph nodes, liver and lungs.

Many carcinoid tumours of the ovary occur in a mature cystic teratoma, in association with gastrointestinal or respiratory type epithelium but a few are pure and not admixed with any other tissues, these being regarded as monophyletic teratomas. Ovarian carcinoid tumours are similar to those that occur in the gastrointestinal tract, usually showing either an insular or a trabecular pattern (Figure 7.50), but are associated with a high incidence of a typical carcinoid syndrome, thus reflecting the ability of these tumours to secrete products directly into the systemic, rather than the portal, circulation.

A strumal carcinoid is a rare neoplasm that combines the features of a struma ovarii and a carcinoid tumour (Figure 7.51). It is thought that the carcinoid component of these neoplasms is derived from the parafollicular cells and that it is thus homologous with the medullary carcinoma of the thyroid gland.

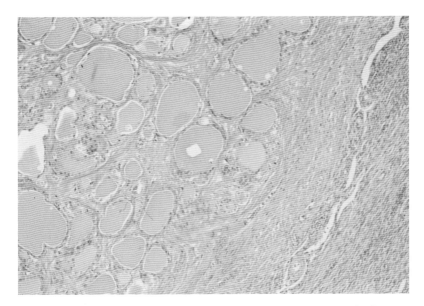

Figure 7.49. Struma ovarii: to the left, the neoplasm is composed of mature thyroid tissue

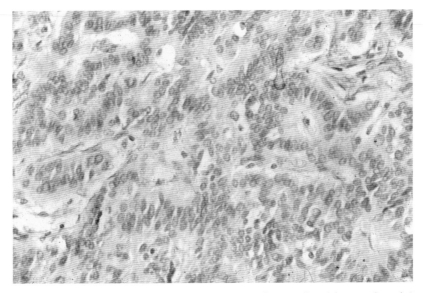

Figure 7.50. Carcinoid tumour of the ovary: uniform cells with round nuclei form trabeculae between which there is fibrous tissue

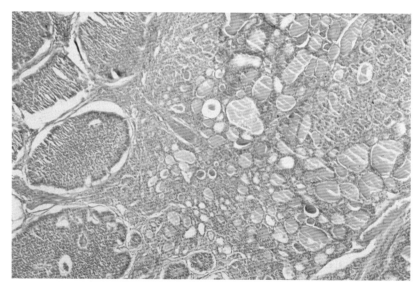

Figure 7.51. Strumal carcinoid tumour of the ovary: to the right, the tumour is composed of thyroid acini containing colloid and to the left, there is insular carcinoid (reproduced with permission from Fox and Buckley, *Atlas of Gynaecological Pathology*, published by MTP Press)

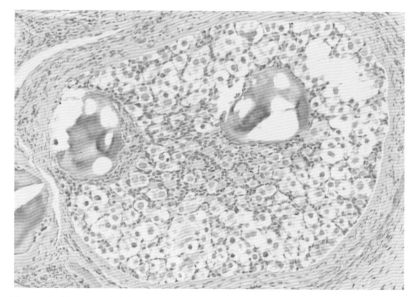

Figure 7.52. Gonadoblastoma of the ovary: the neoplasm is composed of nests of germ cells and sex cord cells set in a dense fibrous stroma; calcification, as seen here, is quite common and may be extensive

Mixed germ cell tumours

Between 5% and 20% of malignant germ cell tumours contain more than one tumour type. A mature teratomatous element does not count in this respect. Such neoplasms occur predominantly in children and young adults. Nearly 50% of stage I tumours treated only surgically recur and so it is usual to give chemotherapy for all except those in which there is only dysgerminoma or grade 1 immature teratoma.

Gonadoblastomas are rare mixed germ cell tumours that are composed of nests of germ cells and sex cord cells surrounded by dense fibrous tissue (Figure 7.52). They are often bilateral and occur predominantly in abnormal gonads: most are detected during investigation of primary amenorrhoea or malformation of the genital tract. The lesions are benign unless there is overgrowth by a malignant germ cell element, most commonly a dysgerminoma and less commonly a yolk sac tumour or embryonal carcinoma.

TUMOURS OF NON-SPECIALISED OVARIAN TISSUE

The only common ovarian tumours of this type are fibromas (see page 156).

MISCELLANEOUS TUMOURS

Steroid cell tumours

Steroid cell tumours are neoplasms which have an endocrine-type architecture and are formed of cells which resemble adrenocortical cells, Leydig cells or luteinised stromal cells. All are thought to derive from the ovarian stroma and may be accompanied by evidence of virilisation. Some of the adrenal-like tumours are associated with clinical features suggestive of Cushing syndrome (Figure 7.53).

Sclerosing stromal tumour

Sclerosing stromal tumours are benign tumours which occur in teenagers and in young women. They are composed of solid, cellular nodules in which there are prominent blood vessels interspersed with hypocellular stroma which may be hyalinised or oedematous (Figure 7.54). Small cysts may be present and some tumours are markedly cystic.

Small-cell carcinoma

Two types of small-cell carcinoma occur in the ovary, both being of unknown origin and nature. Small-cell carcinomas with hyper-

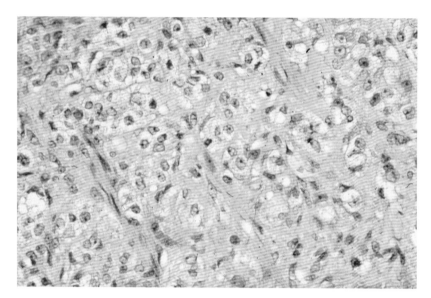

Figure 7.53. Steroid cell tumour of the ovary with an adrenal-like pattern characterised by cells with clear cytoplasm and bland central nuclei

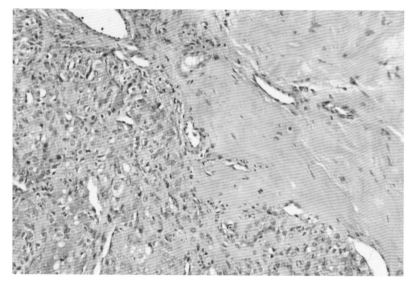

Figure 7.54. Sclerosing stromal tumour of the ovary: to the left is seen one of the solid, cellular nodules with a prominent vascular pattern and to the right, the inter-nodular fibrous tissue which in this case is hyalinised

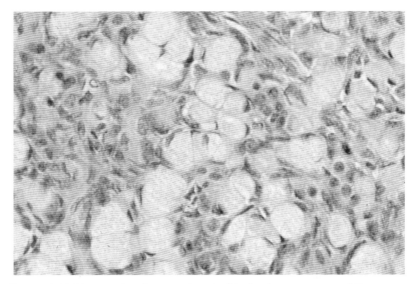

Figure 7.55. Metastatic adenocarcinoma (Krukenberg tumour of the ovary): the fibrous ovarian stroma is infiltrated by large cells with eccentric nuclei and clear cytoplasm (signet-ring cells)

calcaemia are rapidly growing, highly aggressive neoplasms which occur in young women and hypercalcaemia is present in about 50% of cases. These tumours are formed of sheets of small cells, often admixed with larger cells, which show areas of cavitation, haemorrhage and necrosis. The other type of small-cell carcinoma is not associated with hypercalcaemia. It occurs in women of menopausal age, can be bilateral and histologically resembles a small-cell carcinoma of the bronchus.

METASTATIC TUMOURS OF THE OVARY

The ovary is a common site of metastasis, particularly from primary sites in the breast, gastrointestinal tract and uterus. Thus, ovarian metastases are found in approximately one-third of women dying of malignant disease and 10–20% of ovarian tumours which appear originally to be primary to that site eventually turn out to be metastatic in nature.

Ovarian metastases are often bilateral and commonly show extensive areas of haemorrhage and necrosis. Histologically, there tends to be a multinodular pattern and the metastases usually reiterate the appearances of the primary tumour.

A particular form of metastatic ovarian neoplasm is the Krukenberg tumour. These neoplasms are usually bilateral and solid. The metastatic carcinoma cells occur singly, in clumps or sheets, or may form tubules and a proportion are mucus-containing and have their nuclei displaced laterally to give a 'signet-ring' appearance (Figure 7.55). The non-neoplastic stromal cells show a degree of pleomorphism and mitotic activity and are often incorrectly described as having a pseudosarco-matous appearance. Krukenberg tumours are usually metastases from either gastric or colonic carcinomas. The view that gastric carcinomas metastasise to the ovaries by transcoelomic spread is now giving way to the belief that such tumours spread to the ovary via the lymphatics.

Differential cytokeratin (ck) expression can be used immuno-histochemically to distinguish primary epithelial and metastatic ovarian tumours. Primary tumours are usually ck7 positive but ck20 negative.

Endometriosis

Endometriosis is the presence of ectopic endometrial tissue in an extrauterine location. The ectopic tissue occurs most frequently in the ovaries, pouch of Douglas, uterine ligaments, pelvic peritoneum, rectovaginal septum, cervix, appendix, inguinal hernial sacs and the bowel. Foci of endometriosis are occasionally encountered in surgical scars, the vulva, the bladder, the skin or at the umbilicus, and excep-tional instances of lesions occurring in lymph nodes, kidneys, limbs, pleura and lungs have been recorded.

The pathogenesis of endometriosis is still uncertain but one probable mechanism for its development is the reflux of endometrial tissue through the fallopian tubes as a result of retrograde menstruation, with subsequent implantation on, and growth in, the ovaries, pelvic perito-neum and uterine ligaments.

An alternative but not mutually exclusive view is that, in the pelvis at least, endometriosis arises as a result of endometrioid metaplasia of the peritoneal serosa. This is a feasible hypothesis and it may well be that such metaplasia is induced by contact with regurgitated fragments of endometrium. The existence of endometriotic foci in lymph nodes and in distant sites, such as the lung, can clearly not be explained by this mechanism and hence lymphatic or haematogenous dissemination of endometrium must be evoked in such cases. It is almost certain that there is no single pathogenetic mechanism that applies to all cases of endometriosis.

If, however, retrograde menstruation occurs, as is thought to be the case, in most women, the question arises as to why some women develop implants and others do not. There is increasing, although

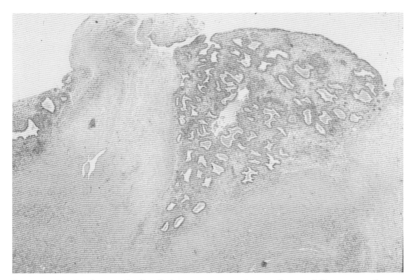

Figure 7.56. Endometriosis of the ovary: on the surface of the ovary there are foci of active endometrium associated with the development of fibrous adhesions

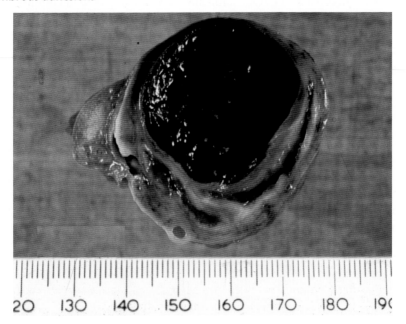

Figure 7.57. 'Chocolate cyst' of the ovary: the cyst contains inspissated blood which has assumed a tarry appearance (reproduced with permission from *The Oxford Textbook of Pathology*, edited by J O'D McGee, P Isaacson and NA Wright, published by Oxford University Press)

largely circumstantial, evidence that immunological malfunction may be involved in this selectivity and there may also be genetic factors.

The pathology of endometriosis is, in essence, simple. The only diagnostic criterion is the presence of histologically recognisable endometrial glands and stroma in an ectopic site (Figure 7.56). Unfortunately, however, the situation is complicated by the tendency towards haemorrhage that is such a characteristic feature of endometriosis. Bleeding into the lesion itself can cause considerable damage and a 'self-destruction' of the endometrial tissue, thus destroying the specific histological findings. Furthermore, haemorrhage into the surrounding tissues releases free iron which is intensely fibrogenic and promotes dense adhesions that tend to obscure the primary lesion.

The early stages of ovarian endometriosis appear to the naked eye as reddish-blue surface implants, which may be raised or dimpled and can measure 1–5 mm across. It is usual for tiny cysts to appear and these progressively enlarge and grow into ovarian tissue, usually reaching a size of 2–5 cm across but occasionally attaining a diameter of up to 10 cm. The cysts have a smooth or granular lining which is brownish-yellow and their walls, originally thin, become eventually thick and fibrotic. Their content of old, semi-fluid or inspissated blood commonly

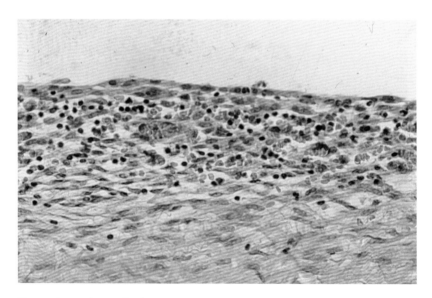

Figure 7.58. The wall of an endometriotic cyst of the ovary: the cyst is lined by non-specific granulation tissue in which there are haemosiderin-containing macrophages and lymphocytes

has a dark brown or black appearance, a feature which has led to the use of the terms 'chocolate' or 'tarry' cyst (Figure 7.57). There is a marked tendency for blood to leak out from endometriotic cysts and this results in the formation of firm adhesions which bind the enlarged ovary down to the posterior surface of either the broad ligament or the uterus. Any attempt at separating the ovary from these structures leads to an escape of brown or black cyst contents. Peritubal adhesions are frequently seen and the tubes may be kinked and distorted. However, the tubal ostia are usually patent and the tubal lumen is rarely obstructed.

The histological diagnosis of ovarian endometriosis is readily made if endometrial glands and stroma are still present in recognisable form in the lesion. It is, however, by no means unusual for the endometrial lining of the cysts either to be so attenuated as to be unrecognisable as such, or to be largely or completely lost. If the endometrial lining has been totally destroyed, the appearance will be that of a simple haemorrhagic cyst lined by granulation tissue and with a fibrous wall in which aggregates of iron-containing macrophages are usually present (Figure 7.58). Under these circumstances, it is justifiable to conclude that the appearances are 'compatible with a diagnosis of endometriosis' or even to make a diagnosis of 'presumptive endometriosis'. It should be noted, however, that in many of these cysts there is no obvious evidence of endometrial stromal tissue and the possibility exists that some are benign endometrioid cystadenomas rather than foci of endometriosis. Any endometrial tissue that is present may show the full range of normal cyclical changes but can appear either to be inactive or to show only proliferative activity. Under the latter circumstances there may be a progression to a simple or atypical hyperplasia.

Extraovarian pelvic endometriosis, for example in the uterosacral and round ligaments, pouch of Douglas, rectovaginal septum or on the surface of the uterus, is seen as multiple bluish-red nodules, patches or cysts, almost invariably with accompanying fibrous adhesions. The lesions are usually small but ligamentous foci may attain a size sufficient to be easily palpable and endometriotic foci in the rectovaginal septum cannot only lead to fixation of the rectum but can extend into the vaginal vault or the rectum to form small haemorrhagic nodules or polyps.

Occasionally, an in situ adenocarcinoma is encountered in an endo-metriotic focus. Overt malignant change gives rise to an endometrioid adenocarcinoma, which is usually of the conventional variety, though any of the many morphological variants of this type of neoplasm, particularly clear-cell adenocarcinomas, can also arise in endometriotic foci. Extra-ovarian endometriosis can also, uncommonly, undergo neoplastic change and give rise to an endometrioid or clear-cell adenocarcinoma in such sites as the uterine ligaments, pouch of Douglas, rectovaginal septum, bladder or colon. Indeed, endometriosis can show the full spectrum of neoplastic change that is seen in the uterine endometrium including stromal sarcoma and mixed tumours. It also has the same propensity to undergo neoplastic change in response to unopposed exogenous estrogen and tamoxifen.

8 Abnormalities related to pregnancy

Ectopic pregnancy

In approximately 1% of all recognised pregnancies, the conceptus implants in a site other than the uterine cavity. The vast majority (95–97%) of such ectopic gestations occur in the fallopian tube. Less common sites are the ovary, cervix and peritoneal cavity and occasional cases of implantation occur in the vagina, liver or spleen.

Tubal pregnancies are predisposed to by any factor which impairs the ability of the tube to transport the fertilised ovum. Hence, congenital abnormalities of the tube, failed tubal sterilisation, the use of a progesterone-only contraceptive pill, salpingitis isthmica nodosa, reconstructive tubal surgery and, most importantly, post-inflammatory tubal damage, are all associated with an increased incidence of tubal pregnancy. In about 50% of such pregnancies the tube is, however, histologically normal. It has been argued that, in such cases, conception occurred during a cycle in which there was delayed ovulation and a short, inadequate luteal phase. Consequently, when the fertilised ovum reached the uterine cavity it had not yet developed to a stage when it was secreting enough human chorionic gonadotrophin (hCG) to prevent decay of the corpus luteum and was flushed back into the tube by a reflux of menstrual blood subsequent to menstrual bleeding. This hypothesis is supported by the fact that tubal gestation occurs only in species which menstruate and by the not uncommon finding of the corpus luteum of pregnancy being on the opposite side to that of a tube containing a pregnancy. This latter phenomenon could, however, also be due to transuterine or transperitoneal migration of the fertilised ovum into the contralateral tube where, because of its relatively advanced stage of development, it implants.

If pregnancy occurs in a woman using an intrauterine contraceptive device, there is a higher than usual risk that it will be ectopically situated. This is not because such a device causes an ectopic pregnancy; it simply fails to prevent extrauterine implantation as effectively as it inhibits implantation within the uterus.

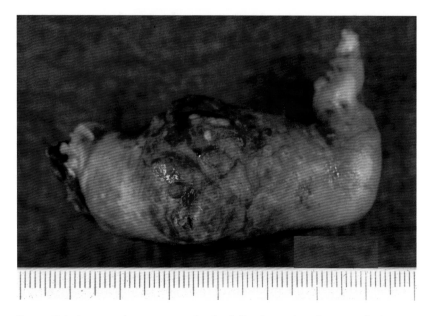

Figure 8.1. An ectopic pregnancy in the fallopian tube: the ampulla is distended and haemorrhagic where trophoblastic tissue has penetrated the full thickness of the tube wall

Within the tube, the fertilised ovum implants most commonly in the ampulla (Figure 8.1). Implantation occurs in exactly the same manner in the tube as it does in the uterus but, nevertheless, a high proportion of tubal pregnancies abort at an early stage. This may be because the conceptus has implanted on the plicae, which offer an inadequate site for placentation, or because trophoblastic invasion of the tubal vessels leads to intramural and intraluminal haemorrhage. Following early miscarriage, the products of conception may be retained in the tube as a form of 'chronic ectopic'; they may be expelled via the uterus or gradually absorbed.

Tubal rupture complicates about 50% of tubal pregnancies and appears to be caused partly by the limited distensibility of the tube and partly to transmural spread of invading extravillous trophoblast with serosal penetration. Rupture is usually acute and is accompanied by intraperitoneal bleeding and the clinical features of an acute abdomen. Less commonly, there is a slow leakage of tubal contents and blood from the tube, which results in a gradually enlarging peritubal haematoma and causes dense adhesions between the tube and surrounding structures such as omentum and intestines. Occasionally, the ureters are obstructed by involvement in this peritubal mass.

Tubal rupture is usually accompanied by fetal death but occasionally the fetus retains sufficient attachment to its blood supply to maintain its viability with the trophoblast growing out through the rupture site and forming a secondary placental site in the abdomen or broad ligament. A secondary abdominal pregnancy of this type may proceed virtually to term.

Gestational trophoblastic disease

The term 'gestational trophoblastic disease' is, by convention, restricted to hydatidiform moles, choriocarcinoma and the placental site trophoblastic tumour.

HYDATIDIFORM MOLE

Only within recent years has it been recognised that there are two fundamentally different types of mole: the complete and partial forms.

Complete hydatidiform mole

Complete moles complicate about one in 1500 gestations in most Western countries but are encountered, for currently unknown reasons, much more frequently in many parts of Africa, Asia and Latin America. They occur particularly in the two extremes of the reproductive era: in women aged less than 18 years or more than 40 years of age and, until relatively recently, used to present either as a miscarriage or as late first-trimester or early second trimester vaginal bleeding. A complete hydatidiform mole, detected at this stage of pregnancy, forms a bulky mass, sometimes weighing as much as 2000 g, which, when in situ, fills and distends the uterine cavity (Figure 8.2). No fetus is present and no normal placental tissue is seen but all the chorionic villi are swollen and distended to give a 'bunch of grapes' appearance. Histologically (Figure 8.3), the villi are devoid of fetal vessels and are markedly oedematous, many showing central liquefaction (cistern formation). A constant feature is atypical growth of the villous trophoblast. Some pleomorphism is often apparent in the proliferating trophoblast but it is the pattern, rather than the degree of proliferation of trophoblastic cells which is atypical, this being either circumferential or multifocal in nature rather than polar, as in the normal first-trimester placenta (Figure 8.4).

This classical clinical picture of complete hydatidiform mole, although still seen in developing countries, is now only rarely encountered in the Western world, where the introduction of routine

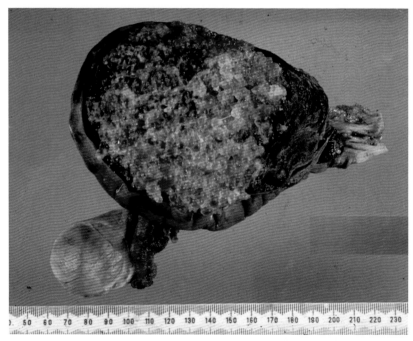

Figure 8.2. A classical complete hydatidiform mole filling and distending the uterine cavity

first-trimester ultrasound scans and the use of transvaginal ultrasound for the investigation of first-trimester bleeding has transformed the clinical features of complete moles. These now most commonly present with ultrasound diagnoses of delayed first-trimester miscarriage or anembryonic pregnancy. The uterus is usually not enlarged, an embryo is not present and, in most cases, the diagnosis of a mole is not made before histological examination. In these early lesions, the typical gross appearances of a complete mole may not be apparent and vesicular villi may not be obvious to the naked eye. There may be, histologically, coexisting hydropic and non-hydropic villi and villi showing frank central cisternal change are often not seen. Those villi which are not vesicular are often branching and have a polypoid or lobulated appearance with mucoid or myxoid change and apoptotic debris in their stroma: fetal vessels are present in many of the villi. Trophoblastic abnormalities are present at this stage but are not as marked as in the classical second-trimester mole; trophoblastic proliferation is usually circumferential rather than multifocal (Figure 8.5).

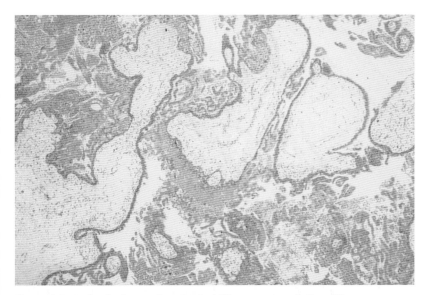

Figure 8.3. A classical complete hydatidiform mole: all the villi are abnormal: there are no fetal vessels; some villi show central cisternal change and there is an abnormal pattern of circumferential perivillous trophoblastic proliferation

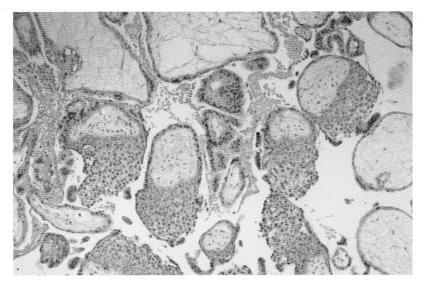

Figure 8.4. Normal first-trimester placental tissue: there is trophoblastic proliferation only at the tips of the villi, in contrast to the circumferential proliferation seen in a molar pregnancy

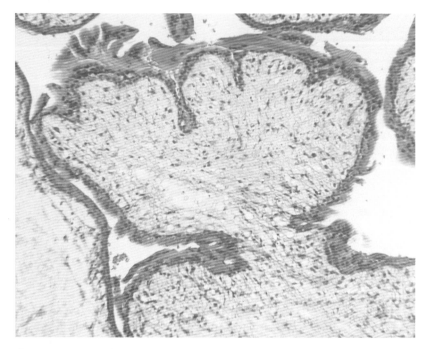

Figure 8.5. An early complete molar pregnancy: villous morphology is polypoid, with irregular trophoblastic proliferation, myxoid stroma and stromal nuclear debris

Cytogenetic studies have shown that 85% of complete hydatidiform moles have a 46XX chromosomal constitution, both X chromosomes being of paternal (androgenetic) origin. It is thought that this is the result of penetration of an anucleate ovum, which then duplicates without cytokinesis. Fifteen percent of complete moles have, however, a 46XY chromosomal constitution, both chromosomes again being derived from the father. It is believed that this type of complete mole results from the entry of two haploid sperms, one X and the other Y, into an abnormal ovum with subsequent fusion and replication. All XY moles are therefore dispermic (or 'heterologous'). It is now clear that, although the vast majority of 46XX moles are monospermic (homozygous), a small proportion resemble the XY moles in being dispermic. This is presumably because of the entry of two, rather than one, haploid X sperms into a defective ovum. p57^{kip2}, the product of a paternally imprinted, maternally expressed gene is not expressed by the villous trophoblast of the androgenic complete mole, which has proved to be a helpful immunohistochemical diagnostic tool.

Hydatidiform moles are a particular form of pregnancy which ends in miscarriage rather than, as is often implied, in a benign neoplasm. Nevertheless, women who have had a complete mole have a much greater risk of subsequently developing a choriocarcinoma (in the region of 2–3%) than do women who have had a normal pregnancy. Attempts have been made to identify those moles most likely to be followed by a choriocarcinoma by grading the degree of trophoblastic hyperplasia. It is maintained that the more marked the degree of trophoblastic proliferation the greater the risk of eventual chorio-carcinoma. Attempts to apply this principle in practice have, however, failed to confirm that the histological features of a complete mole are of any prognostic value. Indeed, reliance upon morphological criteria is potentially dangerous, leading to a false sense of security in some cases and to overtreatment in others. It is now agreed that all women should, after evacuation of a mole, be followed up with serial estimations of hCG levels, surveillance being maintained until, and for up to 1 year after, levels of this placental hormone have returned to normal.

Women in whom hCG values remain elevated or increase during follow-up are classed as having 'persistent trophoblastic disease' or gestational trophoblastic neoplasia. This condition may be attributable to the persistence of residual molar villi or proliferating trophoblast, the development of an invasive mole (see below) or the development of a choriocarcinoma. In most cases, no attempt is made to establish a specific diagnosis and the patients are treated empirically but successfully with a short course of chemotherapy.

Partial hydatidiform mole

Women with a partial hydatidiform mole usually present with late first-trimester vaginal bleeding. In a partial mole, vesicular change affects only a proportion of the villous population of a placenta. The macroscopic appearances are therefore those of a largely normal placenta in which, however, a variable number of distended villi are often, although not invariably, present. Histologically (Figure 8.6), only a proportion of the villi are distended by oedema fluid, these being intermingled with fully normal villi. The scattered vesicular villi have a markedly irregular outline and show atypical trophoblastic proliferation, usually multifocal in nature and commonly less marked than that seen in a complete mole.

The vast majority of partial hydatidiform moles are associated with a fetal triploidy, a small minority having a tetraploid or trisomic chromosomal constitution. Most triploid conceptions do not result in moles and it is now known that if the additional chromosomes are of

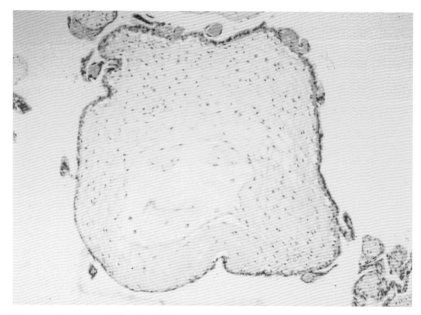

Figure 8.6. A partial hydatidiform mole: the villus is large, contains a central cistern and there are multifocal, circumferential trophoblastic buds; the villi in the lower right of the field are of normal size and appearance

maternal origin a normal placenta will result, whereas if the excess chromosomal load is paternally derived a partial mole will develop. It is now clear that a partial mole can be invasive and can be followed by persistent trophoblastic disease. The relative risk is 0.5% for partial moles compared with 15% for complete moles. Hence, women who have had a partial mole should also be followed up by hCG monitoring.

Invasive hydatidiform mole

In 5–10% of moles, either complete or (rarely) partial, molar villi invade the myometrium, sometimes even penetrating the uterine wall to extend into the broad ligament (Figure 8.7). Myometrial vessels may also be breached by the invasive villous tissue. A deeply invasive mole usually becomes clinically apparent several weeks after apparently complete evacuation of a mole from the uterus, the patient commonly presenting with haemorrhage. Hysterectomy at this stage will reveal intramyometrial haemorrhagic foci and, on microscopy, vesicular villi are seen in the uterine wall and within myometrial vessels. The villous tissue within the vessels can be transported as emboli to sites such as the lung or vagina where they may continue to grow. Any pulmonary

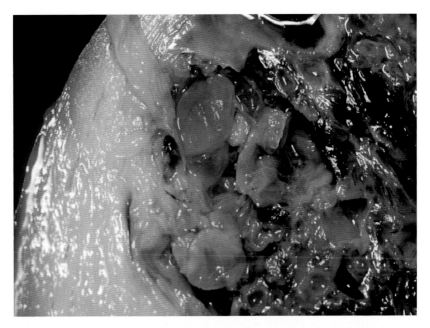

Figure 8.7. Invasive hydatidiform mole: the myometrium is infiltrated by molar tissue, which reaches almost to the uterine serosa

nodules are usually only apparent radiologically but vaginal lesions present as haemorrhagic submucosal nodules. Biopsy of these extrauterine lesions will show molar villi, a finding which excludes a diagnosis of choriocarcinoma.

An invasive mole is not a malignant lesion. Normal placental villi can penetrate deeply into the myometrium, as in the condition of placenta increta, and trophoblastic transportation to extrauterine sites occurs in every pregnancy. An invasive mole simply represents, therefore, a molar version of placenta increta with associated trophoblastic deportation.

In practice, the diagnosis of an invasive mole is now largely obsolete, as women with this type of mole are usually diagnosed as having persistent trophoblastic disease before developing serious complications and are treated by chemotherapy.

CHORIOCARCINOMA

Choriocarcinoma is a malignant neoplasm of trophoblast. It has a unique status because, being of fetal origin, it is the only human tumour which is, in effect, an allograft. Choriocarcinoma is rare in Western countries, complicating approximately one in 45 000 pregnancies, although, as with the hydatidiform mole, it is much more common in many parts of Africa, Asia and South America. Approximately 50% of choriocarcinomas follow a hydatidiform mole, 30% develop after a miscarriage and 20% occur after a normal pregnancy. The time interval between the antecedent pregnancy and the development of a choriocarcinoma is very variable, ranging from a few months to 15 years.

A choriocarcinoma forms single or multiple haemorrhagic nodules within the uterus. These are well delineated and consist of a central area of haemorrhagic necrosis and a peripheral rim of viable tumour tissue. The central necrosis is due to the fact that a choriocarcinoma has no intrinsic blood supply, relying for its oxygenation and nutrition on its ability to invade and permeate the maternal vasculature. Histologically (Figure 8.8), the tumour has a pattern which recapitulates that of the early implanting blastocyst, central cores of cytotrophoblastic cells being surrounded by a peripheral rim of syncytiotrophoblast. The trophoblastic cells do not differ significantly from those of a normal blastocyst and mitotic activity is rarely extensive. Villi are not present in a choriocarcinoma and, indeed, the presence of villous structures refutes this diagnosis. A very rare exception to this is intraplacental choriocarcinoma which arises in the term or near term placenta.

The capacity of malignant trophoblast to invade vessels offers an adequate explanation for the primarily vascular dissemination of this tumour, spread occurring at an early stage to the brain, lungs, liver, kidneys and gastrointestinal tract. It is therefore not surprising that choriocarcinoma was, in the past, a highly lethal neoplasm with a mortality rate little short of 100% and with death occurring in months rather than in years. For no other neoplasm, however, has the advent of chemotherapy more radically altered the prognosis, with over 85% of patients now being permanently cured with cytotoxic drugs.

PLACENTAL SITE TROPHOBLASTIC TUMOUR

Placental site trophoblastic tumour is a neoplasm that originates from the extravillous trophoblastic cells which are normally present in the decidua and myometrium of the placental bed, and form the placental site reaction. A placental site trophoblastic tumour usually occurs after a normal gestation but the neoplasm can also develop after a miscarriage. Symptoms such as abnormal bleeding or amenorrhoea become apparent months or years after the pregnancy.

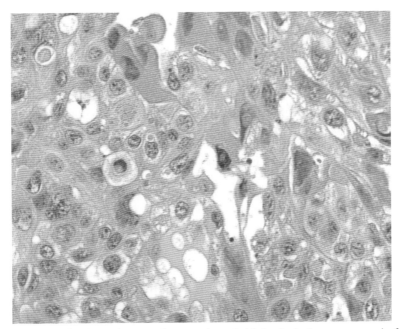

Figure 8.8. Choriocarcinoma: the neoplasm is biphasic, being composed of two types of cell trophoblast: the more darkly-staining syncytiotrophoblast centrally and the paler staining cytotrophoblast

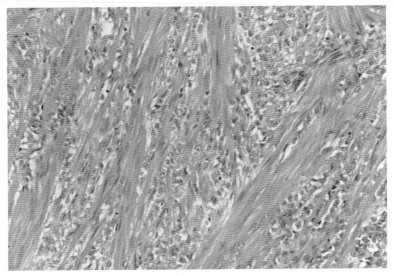

Figure 8.9. Placental site trophoblastic tumour: the tumour is composed of sheets of cells of mononuclear cytotrophoblastic type which infiltrate between the myometrial fibres in sheets and cords

The tumour forms a nodular tan or yellow mass which shows little necrosis or haemorrhage. Histologically (Figure 8.9), trophoblastic cells, predominantly of the mononuclear cytotrophoblastic type, infiltrate between myometrial fibres in sheets, cords and islands. Some multinucleated cells are usually present but the bilaminar pattern of a choriocarcinoma is not seen. Vascular permeation by tumour cells is seen but the massive intravascular growth typical of a choriocarcinoma is not apparent.

Most of these tumours are cured by simple hysterectomy but about 10% extend beyond the uterus and behave in a malignant fashion. In general, neoplasms with an abundance of mitotic figures are most likely to pursue a malignant course but there is no histological feature that can predict malignant behaviour with certainty. Treatment of malignant cases is currently unsatisfactory, for these neoplasms do not respond well to the therapeutic regimen that has met with such success in the treatment of choriocarcinoma.

The related epithelioid trophoblastic tumour behaves clinically like the placental site trophoblastic tumour but is believed to arise from the extravillous trophoblast of the chorion laeve.

Miscarriage

About 15% of recognised pregnancies end, usually during the first trimester, in a spontaneous miscarriage; that is, before the fetus becomes viable. Aetiological factors in miscarriage include infections, uterine abnormalities, endocrine disorders, immunological factors and congenital malformations of the fetus; however, in at least 50% of miscarriages there is a cytogenetic fetal abnormality. Many placentas from miscarried fetuses show either no abnormality or simply changes owing to relatively recent fetal death, such as villous fibrosis; if, however, fetal death occurs at a very early stage of gestation and there is a quite long time lag between fetal demise and delivery, the placenta often shows hydropic change: the villi are markedly oedematous and swollen. Hydropic change in placentas from miscarriages can be confused with a complete hydatidiform mole but, whereas in a mole the trophoblastic mantles of the villi are hyperplastic, in a hydropic miscarriage the villous trophoblast is attenuated (Figure 8.10). Attempts, in cases of miscarriage, to distinguish histologically between placentas from cytogenetically abnormal fetuses and those from cytogenetically normal fetuses have not been successful.

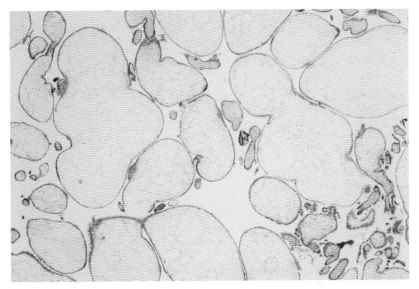

Figure 8.10. Hydropic miscarriage: the villi are oedematous and distended and the covering trophoblast is attenuated; there is no abnormal trophoblastic growth (contrast with Figures 8.3 and 8.6)

Pathology of the placenta

DEVELOPMENTAL ABNORMALITIES

The only common developmental abnormality of the placenta is extrachorial placentation, in which the chorionic plate, from which the villi arise, is smaller than the basal plate, the transition from villous to non-villous chorion taking place not at the placental margin but at some distance inside the circumference of the fetal surface of the placenta (Figure 8.11). If this transition is marked by a flat ring of membranes, the placenta is classed as 'circummarginate' whereas, if this ring has a raised, rolled edge, the placenta is 'circumvallate'. The circummarginate form is devoid of any functional importance and, although circumvallate placentation is associated more frequently than can be explained by chance alone with a rather small baby and, possibly, with a slight excess of congenital malformations, it is not associated with any excess of perinatal mortality. Other aberrant forms of placentation are either relatively common but functionally unimportant, for example the bilobate placenta and accessory lobe, or functionally important but excessively rare, such as placenta membranacea and girdle placenta.

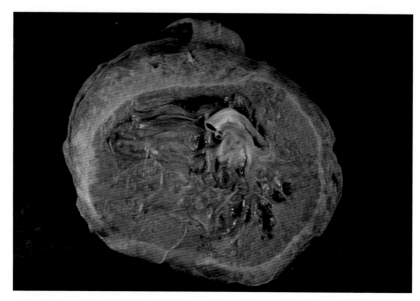

Figure 8.11. Placenta extrachorialis: in this circummarginate placenta, the transition from villous to non-villous chorion takes place inside the circumference of the fetal surface of the placenta and the transition is flat

GROSS LESIONS OF THE PLACENTA

A fresh placental infarct is firm and dark red. As it ages, it becomes progressively harder and its colour changes successively to brown, yellow then white, so that an old infarct appears as an amorphous, hard, white plaque. Histologically, an early infarct is characterised by aggregation of the villi and early necrotic changes in the villous syncytiotrophoblast. With the passage of time, the infarcted villi undergo progressive necrobiosis, so that the old infarct consists only of crowded ghost villi (Figure 8.12).

Small placental infarcts are common and of no importance but extensive infarction, that is necrosis of more than 10% of the placenta, is accompanied by a high incidence of fetal hypoxia, growth restriction and intrauterine death. These ill effects have been thought to be a direct consequence of the loss of viable villous tissue by those who consider that the placenta has little or no functional reserve capacity. However, another common lesion that reduces the number of functioning villi is perivillous fibrin deposition that is sufficiently extensive to appear as either a hard, white plaque or an area of irregular whitish mottling. Histologically, such lesions consist of widely

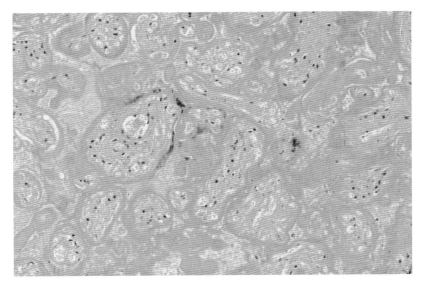

Figure 8.12. An old placental infarct: the villi are visible only as crowded ghost-like structures and the trophoblast has undergone almost complete necrobiosis; this appears grossly as a firm, whitish plaque

separated villi that are entrapped in fibrin, which is filling in and obliterating the intervillous space. The entrapped villi undergo secondary sclerosis but are not infarcted. Nevertheless, they are excluded from playing any role in maternal–fetal transfer and are just as much lost, in a physiological sense, to the fetus as they would be if they were infarcted. Although perivillous fibrin deposition depletes the population of functional villi, this lesion is of no clinical importance, even when it is extensive enough to functionally inactivate 30% of the villi by entrapment in fibrin.

The ability of the placenta to withstand the loss of one-third of its functioning tissue without any discernible effect on fetal growth or development shows that the placenta quite obviously has a considerable functional reserve capacity but it still leaves unexplained why loss of villi due to infarction poses a grave threat to the fetus while a similar, or even greater, loss of villi due to entrapment in fibrin is of no consequence. This paradox is more apparent than real if the pathogenesis of these two lesions is considered. Perivillous fibrin deposition is due to haemodynamic turbulence within the intervillous space, with eddy stasis of maternal blood and laying down of fibrin. Thus, the greater the quantity of maternal blood entering the closed, irregular intervillous space per unit of time, the greater the risk of turbulence and hence of perivillous fibrin deposition. This lesion tends to occur, therefore, in placentas with a particularly good maternal uteroplacental blood flow. Infarction, however, is usually caused by thrombosis of a maternal uteroplacental vessel and therefore extensive infarction implies widespread thrombosis within the maternal vasculature. This would not be expected to occur in a healthy maternal tree and it is therefore no coincidence that extensive infarction is virtually confined to placentas from women with pre-eclampsia, a condition in which an acute 'atherosis' is found in the uteroplacental vessels and which predisposes to thrombosis. Far more importantly, however, in pre-eclamptic women, whether thrombosis occurs or not, there is a severely restricted maternal blood flow to the placenta (the reasons for which are discussed later in this chapter) and it is this limitation of maternal blood flow that is the real cause of the apparent complications of placental infarction.

The true significance of extensive placental infarction is therefore that it is the visible hallmark of a markedly abnormal maternal vasculature and of a severely-restricted materno-uteroplacental blood flow. It is true that under these circumstances the placental infarction may further worsen the situation, but the infarction of itself is not the primary cause of the fetal complications and would be of little or no importance if it occurred in a placenta with an adequate maternal blood supply.

Most other macroscopic lesions of the placenta are of no functional significance and can be ignored. Large retroplacental haematomas, widespread thrombosis of fetal vessels, maternal floor infarction and large haemangiomas can be of clinical importance but these are rare. Otherwise the various plaques, thrombi and cysts that can occur in the placenta lack clinical importance, as does gross placental calcification.

EXTRAVILLOUS TROPHOBLAST AND THE PATHOLOGY OF THE UTEROPLACENTAL VESSELS

It is difficult to accept that most cases of 'placental insufficiency' are caused by intrinsic placental damage and it is becoming increasingly clear that the common factor in most cases of presumed placental inadequacy is a reduced maternal blood flow to the fetoplacental unit. The placenta establishes its own blood supply as a result of invasion of the spiral arteries in the placental bed by extravillous trophoblast which destroys the muscle and elastic tissue of the media of these vessels and replaces these components with fibrinoid material. This process results in the conversion of the thick-walled, muscular spiral arteries into thin-walled, flaccid, sac-like uteroplacental vessels which can passively dilate to accommodate the great increase in maternal blood flow to the placenta which is required as pregnancy progresses. This physiological change within the spiral arteries occurs in two stages. During the first 12 weeks of gestation the extravillous trophoblast invades only the intradecidual portion of the spiral arteries of the placental bed but, after a resting phase, the extravillous trophoblast invades the intramyometrial segments of these vessels between the 14th and 16th weeks of pregnancy.

The factors controlling and limiting intravascular invasion by extravillous trophoblast are not fully understood but involve the interaction of growth factors and their receptors. The crucial importance of this process is shown by the finding that, in women destined to develop pre-eclampsia in the later stages of pregnancy and in many cases of normotensive intrauterine fetal growth restriction, there is a partial failure of placentation, which results in a markedly restricted blood flow to the placenta. This failure has two components. First, while in a normal pregnancy all the spiral arteries in the placental bed are invaded by trophoblast, this process occurs in only a proportion of these vessels in such women, with a significant fraction of the placental bed arteries showing a complete absence of physiological change. Second, in those arteries that are invaded by extravillous trophoblast, the first stage in this process occurs normally with trophoblast evoking physiological changes in their intradecidual segments. There is subsequently a complete failure of the second stage, with endovascular trophoblast failing to advance into the intramyometrial portion of these vessels. Hence, in these women there is an incomplete transformation of the spiral arteries to uteroplacental vessels, an abnormality which has been clearly shown to result in a restriction of the maternal blood flow to the placenta and which will restrict the ability of the mother to provide the fetus with an adequate supply of oxygen and nutrients. A reduced uteroplacental blood flow is, in itself, an adequate cause for all the placental abnormalities seen in pre-eclampsia and for fetal growth restriction. The decreased maternal blood flow also serves as the basis for the maternal syndrome of pre-eclampsia, in so far as a factor appears to be released from the ischaemic placenta which causes widespread maternal endothelial damage.

Most cases of apparent placental insufficiency are, therefore, in reality examples of maternal vascular insufficiency.

PLACENTAL INFECTION

Infective agents may reach the placenta either from the maternal bloodstream to produce a villitis or may ascend from the birth canal to produce a chorioamnionitis.

Villitis may be caused by placental involvement in specific maternal infections, such as rubella, toxoplasmosis, listeriosis (Figure 8.13), syphilis or cytomegalovirus but such conditions account for only a small proportion of cases of villitis, the vast majority of which are of unknown cause. There is a clear association between the presence of a villitis and a high incidence of fetal growth restriction, although the nature of this relationship is obscure. Most cases of villitis are focal, with only a small proportion of the villi showing any evidence of either a healed or an active inflammatory process. This degree of villous damage is unlikely to impair the functional reserve capacity of the placenta and it is possible that the low birth weight in such cases is caused not by villous damage but by infection crossing the placenta and affecting the fetus by inhibiting DNA synthesis. Villitis may thus simply serve as an indicator of possible fetal infection, though it is believed by some to have an autoimmune rather than infective aetiology.

Chorioamnionitis, characterised by polymorphonuclear leucocytic infiltration of the extraplacental and placental membranes (Figure 8.14), is caused by an ascending infection which is commonly of polymicrobial aetiology. Prolonged membrane rupture predisposes to

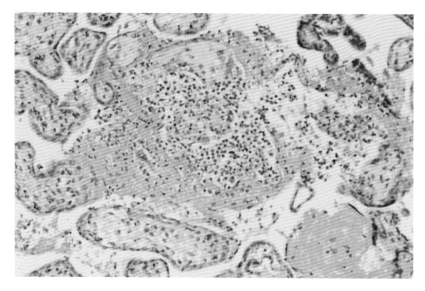

Figure 8.13. Listerial infection of the placenta: there is an acute villitis with abscess formation, destruction of the trophoblast and agglutination of the villi with fibrin deposition

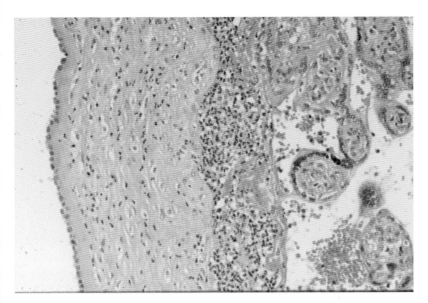

Figure 8.14. Acute chorioamnionitis: the amnion lies to the left and is infiltrated by scanty polymorphonuclear leucocytes but in the chorion and in the subchorionic space, to the right, there is a dense infiltrate of acute inflammatory cells

chorioamnionitis but chorioamnionitis can also occur in the presence of intact membranes. Ascending infections can cause both premature onset of labour and premature rupture of the membranes and chorioamnionitis is a major aetiological factor in preterm labour, particularly before the 35th week of gestation. The mechanism by which an ascending infection stimulates the premature onset of labour is still uncertain but it is thought that cytokines produced by activated macrophages stimulate excess synthesis of prostaglandins, which are of vital importance in initiating parturition, by amniotic and decidual cells. Some cases of preterm delivery associated with an ascending infection are, however, due not to premature onset of labour but to premature rupture of the membranes which may be the result of the combination of release of elastases and collagenases from the neutrophil polymorphonuclear leucocytes infiltrating the membranes and the secretion of proteolytic enzymes by bacteria. In recent years it has been suggested that chorioamnionitis may, because of associated release of cytokines into the fetal circulation, be linked with fetal brain damage; this has not yet, however, been proven.

NON-TROPHOBLASTIC TUMOURS OF THE PLACENTA

The only common non-trophoblastic tumour of the placenta is the haemangioma or 'chorioangioma'. Haemangiomas, usually single but occasionally multiple, are present in 1% of placentas. The vast majority are small and intraplacental where they form well-demarcated, rounded, usually red, intraparenchymal nodules. The uncommon large haemangiomas (Figure 8.15) measuring more than 5 cm in diameter are usually seen as protuberances on the fetal surface of the placenta. Occasionally, they can be found on the maternal surface, where they often appear to replace an entire lobe, or in the membranes attached to the main placental mass only by a vascular pedicle. Histologically, placental haemangiomas have a microscopic appearance identical to that seen in similar tumours elsewhere in the body.

The vast majority of placental haemangiomas are of no clinical importance but a very small minority – those measuring more than 5 cm in diameter – may be associated with a variety of complications that can affect the mother, fetus or neonate. There is a high incidence of polyhydramnios in association with large haemangiomas. The cause of this is obscure but it may precipitate premature labour. Large tumours are also associated, as are multiple small tumours within a single placenta, with an increased incidence of intrauterine fetal hypoxia, fetal growth restriction and intrauterine death. All these complications have been attributed to the fact that a considerable proportion of the fetal blood passes through the tumour, rather than through functional placental tissue, and is therefore returned to the fetus in an unoxygenated and nutrient-poor state. The neonate whose placenta contains a large haemangioma is also subject to a number of complications, usually of a transitory nature, which are a direct consequence of the placental tumour. Prominent among these is cardiomegaly. This is probably a result of the increased fetal cardiac output required for pumping blood through the haemangioma, which in haemodynamic terms can be considered a peripheral arteriovenous shunt. Neonatal oedema is sometimes a manifestation of cardiac failure but can also be due to hypoalbuminaemia which results either from transudation of protein from the surface vessels of the tumour or from chronic fetomaternal bleeding from the haemangioma. Neonatal anaemia can be a result of sequestration of fetal erythrocytes within the tumour, a massive fetomaternal bleed from the haemangioma or a microangiopathic haemolytic anaemia induced by injury inflicted on fetal red blood cells as they transverse the labyrinthine vascular channels of the tumour. Neonatal thrombocytopenia can also be caused by platelet injury within the tumour vessels but is sometimes a manifestation of disseminated intravascular coagulation triggered by a thromboplastic substance released from the haemangioma.

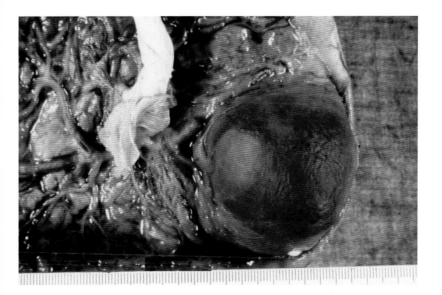

Figure 8.15. Chorioangioma: the chorioangioma, on the fetal surface, at the margin of the placenta forms a well-demarcated dark red, smooth-surfaced mass

THE PLACENTA IN TWIN PREGNANCY (FIGURE 8.16)

Dizygotic twins may have two separate and discrete placentas, each with its own amniotic sac (dichorionic–diamniotic pregnancy). The two placentas may, however, apparently fuse, although there will still be two amniotic sacs. Monozygotic twins may also have separate placentas and amniotic sacs: in some cases there is a single placenta with two amniotic sacs (monochorionic–diamniotic pregnancy) while in others there is a single placenta and a single amniotic sac (mono-chorionic–monoamniotic pregnancy). A distinction between fused dichorionic–diamniotic and monochorionic–diamniotic placentas can be made by examining the septum between the two amniotic sacs (or the T zone at the base of this septum). Chorionic tissue is present between the two layers of the septum in a dichorionic–diamniotic placentation but is absent from the septum of a monochorionic-diamniotic twin placenta (Figure 8.17).

Vascular anastomoses between the twin circulations are often present in diamniotic–monochorionic placentas and these can lead to the twin-to-twin transfusion syndrome in which the recipient twin develops

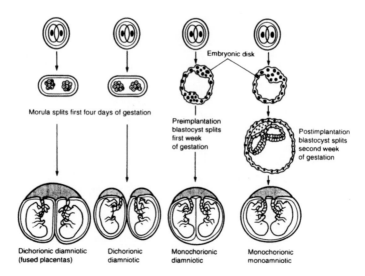

Figure 8.16. Diagrammatic representation of the development and placentation of monozygotic twins

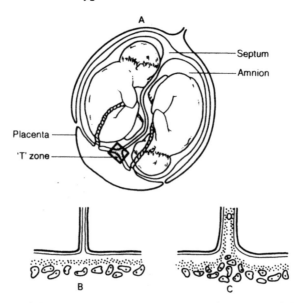

Figure 8.17. (A) Diagrammatic representation of the base of the septum in a diamniotic twin placenta. (B) Diagrammatic representation of the base of the septum in a monochorionic-diamniotic twin placenta: the septum consists of only two layers of amnion. (C) Diagrammatic representation of the base of the septum in a dichorionic-diamniotic twin placenta: chorionic tissue is present in the septum between the two layers of the amnion

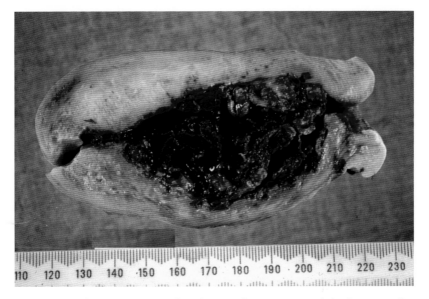

Figure 8.18. Placenta accreta: the placenta has penetrated the lower wall of the uterus and the cavity of the uterus contains retained placental tissue

polyhydramnios and cardiomegaly as a result of vascular overload while the donor twin develops anaemia and oligohydramnios. A transfusion syndrome can lead to the death of the donor twin and such fetal demise can be complicated by brain damage in the surviving twin because of hypovolaemic shock resulting from blood draining into the dead twin's resistance-free vascular bed.

Twin-to-twin transfusion rarely occurs in monochorionic-monoamniotic placentas but entanglement of the cords leads to a high fetal mortality in this form of twin placentation.

PLACENTA ACCRETA

This condition is characterised by abnormal adherence, either in whole or in part, of the placenta to the underlying uterine wall. The pathological basis for this undue tenacity is thought to be a complete or partial absence of the decidua basalis. A placenta accreta is now regarded as being one in which the placental villi adhere to, invade into or penetrate through the myometrium. If the placental villi are attached to the myometrium (Figure 8.18) but do not invade the muscle, it is classed as placenta accreta. If the villi invade the myometrium it is known as placenta increta, while, if the villi penetrate through the full thickness of the myometrium, the stage of `placenta percreta' has been reached A placenta percreta may invade adjacent tissues such as the bladder.

Placenta accreta occurs most commonly in women with a placenta praevia and a history of a previous caesarean section. The condition is characterised by a failure of separation of the placenta in the third stage of labour and, if the placenta is only partially of the accreta type, there may also be severe bleeding.

9 Cervical and other gynaecological cytology

Cervical cytology

Worldwide, comprehensive, quality assured population screening by microscopic examination of cellular material obtained from the cervix has significantly reduced the incidence of and mortality from invasive cervical carcinoma. It has been estimated that cytology-based population screening has prevented up to 4500 deaths a year in England: it is a simple, safe and inexpensive method of detecting cervical premalignancy. Provided that the sample is correctly taken and is interpreted with skill and care, it will provide the general practitioner or gynaecologist with reliable information about the state of the cervix and enable them to reassure the woman about her risk of cervical neoplasia with a high degree of confidence.

INDICATIONS FOR A CERVICAL CYTOLOGY TEST

There are two indications for taking a cervical cytology sample:
- population screening for cervical precancer and early cervical cancer

- as part of the follow-up after treatment of cervical neoplasia.

Population screening

Worldwide, there are nearly half a million new cases of cervical carcinoma a year, of which over 75% occur in developing countries, where at best cervical screening is opportunistic and a cervical cytology test is only available on request. By contrast, in many developed countries, screening healthy women for preinvasive and early invasive cancer of the cervix is highly organised and well women are invited at regular intervals to attend for a cytology test. The intervals between cytology tests affect the protective value of the test (Table 9.1), from which it can be seen that the shorter the interval between tests, the greater the protection afforded to the woman.

Table 9.1 Incidence of squamous cell carcinoma of the cervix following two or more normal cytology tests, as a proportion of the incidence in a comparable unscreened population

Time since last smear (months)	Proportional incidence
0–11	0.06
12–23	0.08
24–35	0.12
36–47	0.19
48–59	0.26
60–71	0.28
72–119	0.63
120+	–1.00

In countries with organised screening programmes, such as the UK, Denmark and the Netherlands, the interval between tests is 3 or 5 years. The frequency of screening in these countries is largely determined by the resources available for the screening programme. Where resources are limited, it has been found that screening every 5th year with a compliance rate of 80% is a much more effective way of reducing cancer mortality and morbidity than annual or 3-yearly screening of a small proportion of women at risk.

The target population can only be defined in terms of age. Attempts to define 'at risk' groups using other parameters, such as smoking habits or sexual activity, are theoretically appealing but impossible to implement in clinical practice. In England, a cervical cytology test is offered every 3 years to all women aged 25–49 years and every 5 years to women aged 50–64 years. Cervical cytology ceases in women with a negative (normal) screening history at the age of 65 years. This policy, introduced in 2004, is predicted to prevent 63% of cervical cancers in women aged 20–79 years compared with an unscreened population. Further reductions in cervical cancer incidence could be achieved by increasing the sensitivity of the screening test (see below) or extending screening to older women. In contrast to previous practice, there is no justification for taking a second cytology test 1 year after the first negative test or additional tests when a women is starting oral contraceptive therapy, having an intrauterine contraceptive device inserted, is pregnant, has genital warts or herpes or admits to being a heavy smoker, provided that the woman is asymptomatic, is participating in the routine screening programme and has had a negative test within the previous 3–5 years. However, women who are HIV positive should be screened annually, as they are recognised to have a higher incidence of cervical neoplasia.

Follow-up after treatment of cervical neoplasia

Cervical cytology tests are mandatory in monitoring women who have been treated for cervical intraepithelial neoplasia (CIN) or cervical glandular intraepithelial neoplasia (CGIN). It is possible, by cervical cytology, to detect residual disease due to incomplete clearance following ablative or excisional treatment and also to detect recurrent disease. Current National Health Service Cervical Screening Programme guidance is that women treated for high grade disease (CIN2, CIN3 or CGIN) require 6- and 12-month cytology and annual cytology for the subsequent 9 years before returning to screening at the routine interval (3 or 5 years depending on the woman's age). Women treated for low grade disease (CIN1 and viral condyloma) require follow-up cytology at 6, 12 and 24 months and, if all the tests are negative, they may then revert to screening at the routine interval. However, there is accumulating evidence that testing for high-risk types of human papillomavirus (HPV) is more sensitive than cytology in detection of residual or recurrent cervical neoplasia after treatment and it is likely that in the future HPV testing will replace cytology in follow up of women after treatment for CIN or CGIN (see below).

SPECIMEN COLLECTION

The cervical cytology test is based on the knowledge that neoplastic cells lose the cohesive properties of normal cells and are therefore readily dislodged when the cervix is scraped. In practice, the earliest and smallest neoplastic lesion can be detected by examination of the cytology before it is visible to the naked eye. Thus, cytological investigation can provide a very sensitive method of detecting neoplasia.

Several methods have been described for obtaining cytological samples from the uterine cervix and the device used depends on whether one is preparing a conventional cervical smear or a liquid-based cytology (LBC) preparation. Irrespective of the sampling method used, it is essential that material is obtained from the transformation zone, the area in which the majority of the precursors of cervical cancer arise. The equipment required includes gloves; specula in a range of sizes; the appropriate sampling device; slides, fixative, pencil and slide carrier for conventional cytology tests; or vials and a ball point pen for LBC preparations (Figure 9.1).

The cervical cytology sample is obtained under direct vision with the vaginal speculum in position and the woman in the left-lateral or dorsal position. Good illumination of the cervix is essential and a speculum of suitable size should be used. The sample should be taken before bimanual examination of the cervix to prevent bleeding and before the

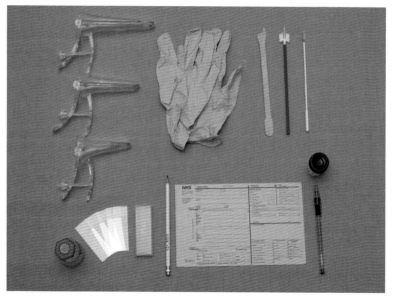

Figure 9.1. Equipment required for taking a cervical cytology sample

application of acetic acid if the cytology test is taken at colposcopy. Lubricant apart from water should be avoided or used very sparingly and the cervix must be clearly visualised before the cytology test is taken. It should not be wiped or cleansed in any way prior to sampling.

Sampling devices

The three types of sampling device in common use: the cervical spatula, endocervical brush and cervical broom, are illustrated in Figure 9.2. Three methods are recommended (Figure 9.3):

- extended tip (Aylesbury) spatula alone

- cervical broom

- combination of a spatula for the ectocervical sample and the endocervical brush for the endocervical sample.

An endocervical brush should never be used alone.

In all cases, it is essential that the material for conventional cytology tests is spread and fixed as quickly as possible to prevent air drying, which will distort cellular detail and will hamper accurate interpretation in the laboratory. Cytological specimens from postmenopausal women and bloodstained cytological specimens are particularly prone to dry very rapidly.

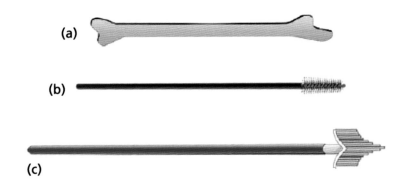

Figure 9.2. Sampling devices: (a) combined spatula with an Aylesbury end (extended tip, right) and an Ayre end (left); (b) endocervical brush; (c) cervical broom (reproduced with permission from *Cytopathology* 2007;18:133–9)

The material from the sampling devices is fixed in a similar manner whichever of these methods is used for its collection. Having been spread as quickly as possible, the material is fixed by flooding the slide with fixative from a dropper bottle, spraying the slide with an aerosol fixative or immersion of the slide in a container of fixative. In all cases, the fixative of choice is 95% ethyl alcohol. The slide should be fixed for at least 10 minutes and then removed from the fixative and placed dry in a slide box for transportation.

Preparing a liquid-based cytology sample

LBC samples are obtained in the same way as conventional cytology tests but only plastic sampling devices should be used and the manufacturer's instructions for collecting the sample must be carefully followed. This is because the protocol for rinsing the sample into the vial of collection fluid depends on the system used.

After completing the procedure, the request form should be completed to include the woman's surname, forename, postal address and date of birth, specimen type (conventional or LBC), clinical appearance of the cervix, relevant symptoms, menstrual history and current methods of contraception. Details of the cervical cytology history and date of the last test should also be provided, if available.

An excellent illustrated account of the technique for obtaining cervical cytology samples is available from the British Society for Clinical Cytology (BSCC) in both video and booklet formats.[1]

Device	Method
Extended tip spatula	The end of the spatula most appropriate to the anatomy of the portio should be used (Figure 9.2). For nulliparae, this is usually the Aylesbury end and for multiparae the broader Ayre end. It is important that the spatula is kept in firm contact with the cervical surface whilst it is rotated through at least 360 degrees (a).
(a) 360°	The material from the spatula is spread on to a glass slide as quickly as possible, using longitudinal sweeps to ensure that material from both sides of the spatula is taken.
Combined spatula and endocervical brush	The spatula sample is obtained as described above. The endocervical brush is inserted into the endocervical canal so that the lower bristles are still visible and then rotated gently through 180 degrees (b).
(b) 90°–180°	The material from the brush is transferred to a glass slide by rolling the brush over the outer third of the slide in the opposite direction from that used to collect the sample. The material from the spatula is then spread on the central third of the same slide. Alternatively, the brush and spatula samples can each be spread on half the slide.
Cervical broom	The tip of the broom is inserted into the external os and the broom rotated through 360 degrees at least five times, applying gentle pressure by rolling the handle clockwise between thumb and forefinger. The cellular sample is spread on a glass slide by sweeping first one side of the brush down the slide and then the second side of the brush.

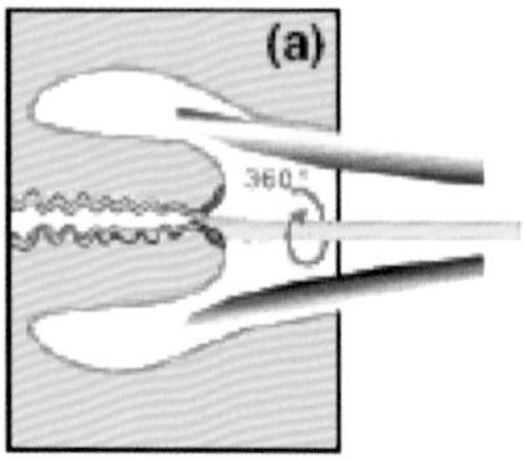

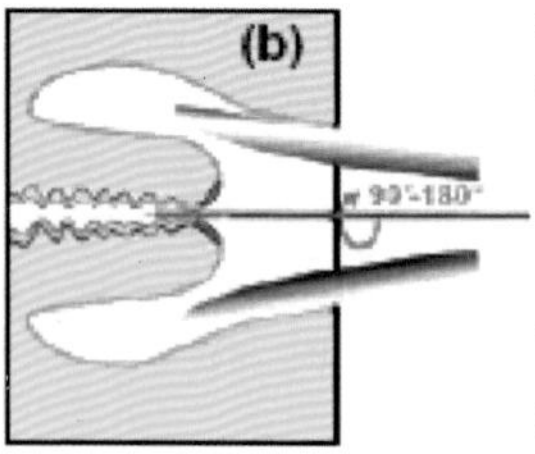

Figure 9.3 Sampling and preparing a conventional smear

PREPARATION AND INTERPRETATION OF CERVICAL SAMPLES

It is important for the gynaecologist to be aware of the procedures for processing cervical samples once they arrive at the laboratory.

Conventional smears

Conventional smears are stained with the Papanicolaou stain, which is designed to display epithelial cell morphology and permits visualisation of the nucleus and cytoplasm of the cell. Staining may be carried out on an automated staining machine or manually. In either event, the nuclear chromatin and nuclear membrane should be crisp and clearly defined and the chromatin stained a blue-black colour. The cytoplasm should stain a delicate blue or pink. Nuclear cytoplasmic ratios are important features for the cytologist, since alteration of the normal ratios is an indication that the cells may be neoplastic.

The Papanicolaou stain has another valuable property, in that it does not affect the transparency of the cytoplasm, so it is possible to examine clumps of cells in conventional smears as well as single discrete cells. The stain also provides information about the type of epithelial cells present in the smear. For example, squamous epithelial cells have a dense cyanophilic or eosinophilic cytoplasm, whereas glandular cells have very delicate cytoplasm. Cells which are highly keratinised (such as those found in invasive squamous carcinomas) have bright orange cytoplasm. Thus, the colour and shape of the cells are important diagnostic features for the cytologist and these will only be preserved if the smears are properly prepared and fixed without drying. Once the smear has been stained, it is dehydrated and mountant and a coverslip applied. It can now be examined under a microscope.

Liquid based cytology samples

LBC samples are processed to remove as much as possible of the non-epithelial component (mucus, red blood cells and inflammatory cells) by either density gradient sedimentation (SurePath™, Beckton Dickinson & Co.) or membrane filtration (ThinPrep®, Hologic) and the resulting epithelial cell component placed on a glass slide as a circular deposit, which is stained and coverslipped as described above.

Examining the cytology preparations

The primary screener examines the cells field by field, searching for the occasional abnormal cell amid the numerous normal cells. If no abnormality is encountered, the primary screener may prepare and issue the report. If abnormality is suspected the smear or LBC preparation is passed to a supervisory biomedical scientist for a second opinion. If the biomedical scientist thinks that abnormal cells are present the smear or LBC preparation is passed to an advanced biomedical scientist practitioner or pathologist for reporting.

Screening is a labour-intensive task which requires a high level of skill and concentration. All laboratories have in place a quality control system which is designed to minimise the risk of overlooking an abnormal specimen. This is achieved in most countries by the supervisor checking a random ten percent 10% of specimens judged to be negative by primary screeners but in the UK it is achieved by 'rapid review' or 'rapid preview' of all negative specimens. Other quality control measures include:

- monitoring the workload of primary screening staff, advanced practitioners and pathologists

- calculation of the sensitivity and positive predictive value for detection of high-grade disease for individuals and laboratories

- retrospective review of cytology tests of women who develop intraepithelial or invasive cervical neoplasia with a history of negative cytology tests

- cytological/histological/colposcopic correlation in women with an abnormal cytology test report.

COMPONENTS OF A CERVICAL CYTOLOGY SAMPLE

The normal cells that can be recognised in a cervical cytology specimen are itemised below and include (Figures 9.4 to 9.8):

- squamous epithelial cells from the ectocervical epithelium

- metaplastic squamous epithelial cells from the transformation zone

- endocervical cells (also known as glandular or columnar cells) from the endocervical canal

- epithelial and stromal cells from the endometrial cavity, red blood cells and inflammatory cells.

In addition, Döderlein bacilli, mucus strands and spermatozoa may be seen. A number of specific infections can be identified, for example, *Candida* species, *Trichomonas vaginalis*, bacterial vaginosis, *Actinomyces*-like organisms, HPV infection (koilocytes) and genital *Herpes simplex* virus infection (Figures 9.9 to 9.11). The cytology specimen also reflects the hormonal status of the woman, in that tests taken from women with high levels of circulating estrogen contain numerous large

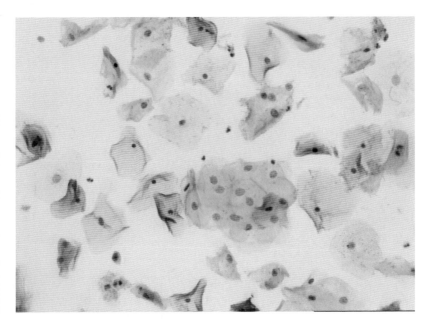

Figure 9.4. Normal cervical squamous epithelial cells

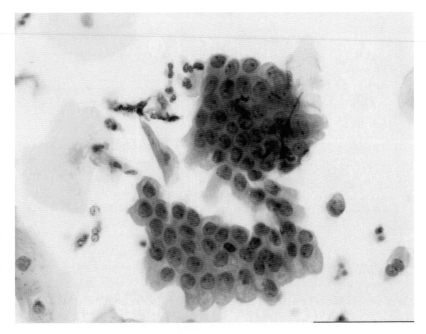

Figure 9.5. Normal endocervical cells

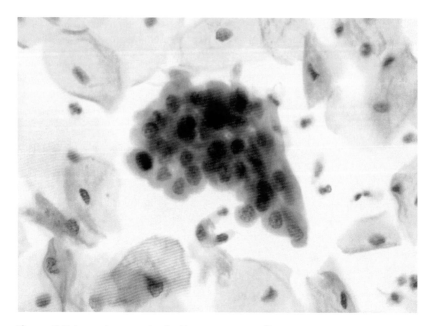

Figure 9.6. Immature metaplastic squamous cells

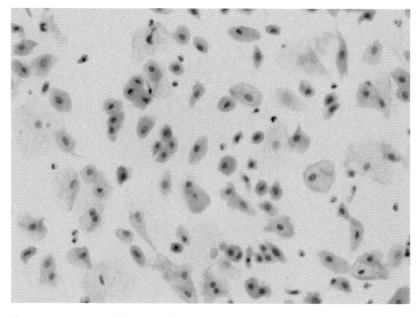

Figure 9.7. An atrophic cervical sample; it is relatively poorly cellular and composed largely of basal and parabasal cells

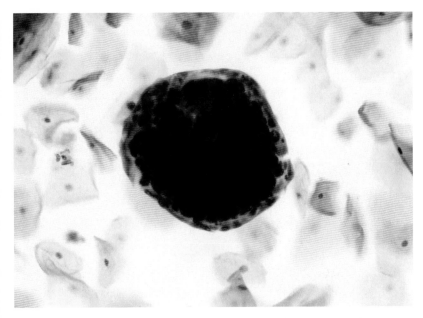

Figure 9.8. Endometrial cells: stromal cells surrounded by a rim of epithelial cells in a characteristic 'top hat' configuration

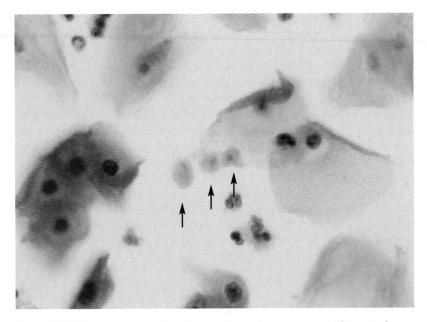

Figure 9.9. *Trichomonas vaginalis*: pear-shaped organisms with central polar bodies (arrowed) associated with an intermediate squamous cell

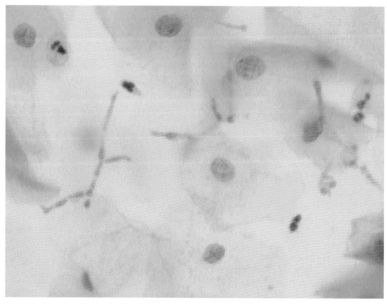

Figure 9.10. Candida: branching septate fungal hyphae and spores associated with intermediate squamous epithelial cells

superficial squamous cells, whereas tests taken from a postmenopausal women will be composed of small squamous cells with an atrophic appearance, often described as 'parabasal cells' (Figure 9.7).

Neoplastic cells thought to be derived from precancerous squamous or glandular lesions are described as dyskaryotic and are recognised by their abnormal nuclei. These are irregular in size and shape, usually dark staining (hyperchromatic) and enlarged, resulting in an increased nuclear–cytoplasmic ratio and have abnormal chromatin granularity and distribution (Figures 9.12, 9.13 and 9.15). In addition, several features suggest that dyskaryotic squamous cells are derived from squamous cell carcinoma of the cervix rather than CIN. Cells from cervical squamous carcinoma are usually highly keratinised and vary greatly in shape and size (Figure 9.14) Moreover, cytological features may suggest that the neoplastic lesion is glandular rather than squamous and may suggest the likely site of origin: endocervical, endometrial or extrauterine (Figure 9.15).

THE CYTOLOGY TEST REPORT

The report should be provided in narrative form and contain the following information:

● whether the specimen is adequate for reporting

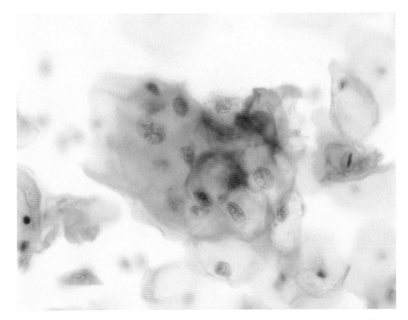

Figure 9.11. Koilocytes showing borderline nuclear change: these cells have the characteristic perinuclear halo with a sharply defined outer margin; there is minimal nuclear abnormality insufficient to warrant a diagnosis of mild dyskaryosis; compare with Figure 9.12

- a description of the cells seen and the histological lesion predicted
- guidance on further management.

The terminology used to report cervical cytology tests in the UK is shown in Table 9.2. An equivalent terminology (the Bethesda system), in use in the USA and several other countries, is shown in Box 9.2 and Table 9.3. The Bethesda system differs from the UK system in that it introduces a two-tier rather than a three-tier grading system for reporting squamous dyskaryosis, namely high- and low-grade squamous intraepithelial lesions (HSIL and LSIL), and atypical squamous (or glandular) cells (ASCUS or AGUS), corresponding to borderline change in the BSCC system. All cytological changes consistent with HPV infection are reported as LSIL whereas in the UK koilocytes showing only slight nuclear atypia due to HPV infection are considered to show borderline changes. It is likely that BSCC terminology will also shortly move to a two-tier system of low- and high-grade dyskaryosis (Table 9.3).

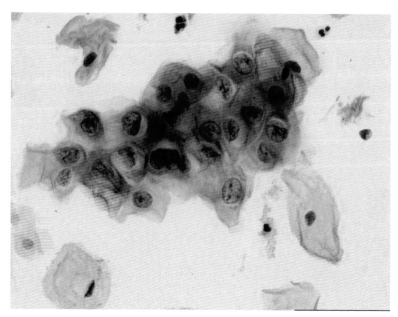

Figure 9.12. Mild dyskaryosis: the abnormal nuclei occupy less than half the area of the affected cells

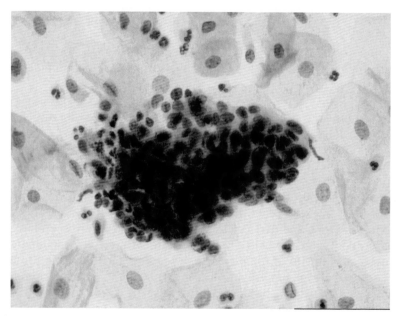

Figure 9.13. Severe dyskaryosis: a group of crowded disorganised cells in which abnormal nuclei occupy virtually all of each of the affected cells

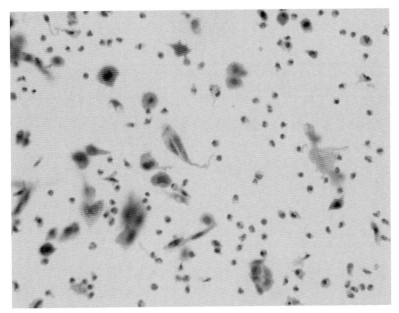

Figure 9.14. Squamous cell carcinoma: large abnormal keratinised cells, fibre and tadpole-shaped cells and inflammatory cells associated with fragments of necrotic debris are highly suggestive of the presence of squamous cell carcinoma

INTERPRETATION OF THE CERVICAL CYTOLOGY TEST REPORT

The inadequate (unsatisfactory) cervical cytology test

Conventional cervical smears may be reported as inadequate for a number of reasons (Figure 9.16):

- the degree of cellularity is judged to be insufficient, taking account of the woman's age and hormonal status

- it is composed entirely of superficial squamous cells, suggesting that the vagina rather than the cervix has been sampled

- it is poorly fixed or air dried

- the cellular material is so thickly spread that the epithelial cells cannot be evaluated

- the epithelial cells are obscured by blood, menstrual debris, inflammatory cells, bacteria or spermatozoa and cannot be evaluated

- it is composed entirely of endocervical cells, unless the only purpose of the test was to sample the endocervical mucosa.

Table 9.2 Interpretation and management of cytology test results (based on BSCC terminology and NHSCSP guidelines)

Cytology report	Explanation	Action
Inadequate	Insufficient epithelial cellular material	Repeat sample as soon as convenient
	Specimen composed entirely of superficial squamous cells or endocervical cells	Refer for colposcopy after three consecutive inadequate samples
	Inadequate fixation	
	Epithelial cells largely obscured by blood, menstrual debris, inflammatory cells, bacteria or spermatozoa	
	Thickly spread cellular material	
Negative	No atypical, dyskaryotic or malignant cells identified	Routine recall
Borderline changes	Sample in which there is doubt whether the nuclear changes are due to inflammation or neoplasia	Repeat sample in 6 months after one test reported as borderline change in squamous cells
		Refer for colposcopy after three consecutive samples reported as borderline change in squamous cells or three samples reported as borderline change in squamous cells in a 10-year period
		Refer for colposcopy after one test reported as borderline change in endocervical cells
Mild dyskaryosis	Squamous cellular changes consistent with origin from CIN1	Ideally, refer for colposcopy but repeat sample in 6 months acceptable
Moderate dyskaryosis	Squamous cellular changes consistent with origin from CIN2	Refer for colposcopy
Severe dyskaryosis	Squamous cellular changes consistent with origin from CIN3	Refer for colposcopy
Severe dyskaryosis ? invasive carcinoma	Squamous cellular changes consistent with origin from CIN3 but with additional features that suggest the possibility of squamous carcinoma	Urgent referral for colposcopy
? glandular neoplasia	Cellular changes suggestive of neoplasia in the endocervix, endometrium, adnexae or peritoneum	Urgent referral for colposcopy or gynaecological opinion, depending on the predicted site of the lesion (endocervix or elsewhere)

Box 9.2 The 2001 Bethesda System: terminology for reporting results of cervical cytology

SPECIMEN TYPE
Indicate conventional smear versus liquid based preparation versus other.

SPECIMEN ADEQUACY
Satisfactory for evaluation.
Unsatisfactory for evaluation … *(specify reason).*

GENERAL CATEGORISATION (OPTIONAL)
Negative for intraepithelial lesion or malignancy.
Other: see 'Interpretation/result' *(i.e., endometrial cells in a woman ≥ 40 years of age).*
Epithelial cell abnormality: see 'Interpretation/result' *(specify 'squamous' or 'glandular' as appropriate).*

INTERPRETATION/RESULT
NEGATIVE FOR INTRAEPITHELIAL LESION OR MALIGNANCY

ORGANISMS
Trichomonas vaginalis.
Fungal organisms morphologically consistent with *Candida* spp.
Shift in flora suggestive of bacterial vaginosis.
Bacteria morphologically consistent with *Actinomyces* spp.
Cellular changes consistent with herpes simplex virus.

OTHER NON-NEOPLASTIC FINDINGS (optional to report; list not inclusive)
Reactive cellular changes associated with:
• inflammation (includes typical repair)
• radiation
• intrauterine contraceptive device.
Glandular cells status post-hysterectomy.
Atrophy.

OTHER
Endometrial cells *(in a woman ≥ 40 years of age).*

EPITHELIAL CELL ABNORMALITIES

SQUAMOUS CELL
Atypical squamous cells:
• of undetermined significance (ASCUS)
• cannot exclude HSIL (ASC-H).
Low-grade squamous intraepithelial lesion (LSIL) *(encompassing: HPV/mild dysplasia/CIN 1).*
High-grade squamous intraepithelial lesion (HSIL) *(encompassing: moderate and severe dysplasia, carcinoma in situ; CIN2 and CIN3)*
• *with features suspicious for invasion.*
Squamous cell carcinoma.

GLANDULAR CELL
Atypical:
• endocervical cells (not otherwise specified *or specify in comments*)
• endometrial cells (not otherwise specified *or specify in comments*)
• glandular cells (not otherwise specified *or specify in comments*).
Atypical:
• endocervical cells, favour neoplastic
• glandular cells, favour neoplastic.
Endocervical adenocarcinoma in situ.
Adenocarcinoma:
• endocervical
• endometrial
• extrauterine
• not otherwise specified.

OTHER MALIGNANT NEOPLASMS: *(specify).*

Table 9.3 Comparison of the existing British Society for Clinical Cytology (BSCC) terminology, proposed new BSCC terminology and the Bethesda System

BSCC 1986	Proposed New BSCC terminology	Bethesda system 2001
Negative	Negative	Negative for intraepithelial lesion or malignancy
Inadequate	Inadequate	Unsatisfactory for evaluation
Borderline nuclear change	1. Borderline change, high-grade dyskaryosis not excluded 2. Borderline change in endocervical cells 3. Borderline change, squamous but not otherwise specified.	1. Atypical squamous cells (ASC) ASCUS (undetermined significance) ASCH (cannot exclude HSIL) 2. Atypical endocervical/ endometrial/glandular cells: NOS or favour neoplastic
Mild dyskaryosis	Low-grade dyskaryosis (includes all cases of koilocytosis provided that no high-grade dyskaryosis is present)	Low-grade squamous intraepithelial lesions (LSIL)
Moderate dyskaryosis Severe dyskaryosis	High-grade dyskaryosis	High-grade squamous intraepithelial lesions (HSIL)
Severe dyskaryosis ? invasive	Severe dyskaryosis/? invasive	Squamous cell carcinoma

? Glandular neoplasia	? Glandular neoplasia:
	    Endocervical
	    Non-cervical
		1. Endocervical carcinoma in situ
		2. Adenocarcinoma:
		    Endocervical
		    Endometrial
		    Extrauterine
		    NOS

LBC samples are inadequate if there are insufficient numbers of squamous epithelial cells present. Both types of cervical cytology test are reported as inadequate if endocervical cells are not identified in a test taken for follow up of an endocervical glandular abnormality. They will also be reported as inadequate if the specimen taker indicates on the request from that the cervix has not been completely visualised, unless abnormal cells are identified, in which case they will be reported according to the degree of abnormality present.

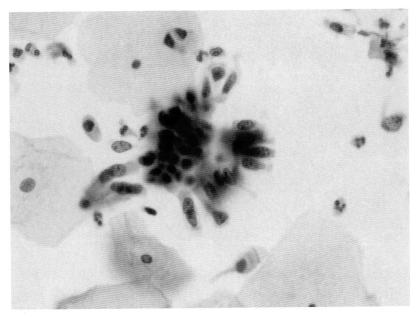

Figure 9.15. Endocervical adenocarcinoma in situ: a group of dyskaryotic endocervical cells showing rosette formation, nuclear overlapping, pseudostratification and feathering; compare with Figure 9.5

Negative

The majority of cytology tests are reported as negative, indicating that dyskaryotic cells have not been identified. However, other information about the specimen which may be useful for the clinician in his or her management of the woman's condition should be reported, including, for example, information about specific infection, such as trichomonas or candida, or the presence of endometrial cells in a specimen from a postmenopausal woman or woman aged more than 40 years.

Mild, moderate and severe dyskaryosis

Cytology tests containing cells showing varying degrees of squamous dyskaryosis indicate the presence of CIN. The grade of dyskaryosis is determined from the nuclear–cytoplasmic ratio assessed by comparing the area of the nucleus with the area of the affected cell. In mild dyskaryosis, the nucleus occupies less than half the area of the cell, in moderate dyskaryosis the nucleus occupies between half and two-thirds of the area of the cell and in severe dyskaryosis more than two-thirds of the area of the cell. Mild dyskaryosis is suggestive of origin

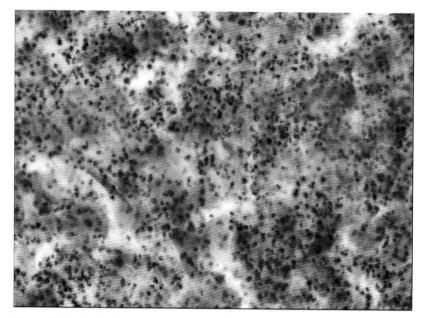

Figure 9.16. An inadequate conventional cervical smear in which the epithelial cells are almost totally obscured by polymorphs

from CIN1, moderate dyskaryosis suggestive of origin from CIN2 and severe dyskaryosis suggestive of origin from CIN3. The most severe degree of dyskaryosis is reported and should always be regarded as indicative of the lowest grade of CIN likely to be present.

Severe dyskaryosis/invasive squamous carcinoma

It should be remembered that cytology involves the examination of cells shed from the surface layers of the epithelium lining the ecto- and endocervix and a definitive diagnosis of actual invasion of the sub-epithelial connective tissue by neoplastic cells cannot be made on the cytology test. Thus, the cytology report can only provide a provisional diagnosis which requires confirmation by biopsy. Despite this limitation, experienced cytopathologists can be remarkably accurate in their prediction as to whether a lesion is invasive or intraepithelial and a cytological diagnosis of possible invasion should not be ignored.

Cytologists have to be aware of the effect of radiotherapy or cytotoxic drug therapy on the cervical epithelium. These forms of therapy produce changes very similar to dyskaryosis and may lead to misinterpretation of the cytology test. Cytology tests taken within 3 months of laser ablation or biopsy often contain atypical cells. It is important for the cytologist to be given a full clinical history to minimise the risk of such mistakes. Women on hormone replacement therapy often have a proliferative pattern with abundant endocervical cells, which can be misleading unless the clinical history is known.

Glandular neoplasia

Samples with cytological features suggestive of CGIN or invasive endocervical, endometrial or extrauterine adenocarcinoma, are reported as '?glandular neoplasia' with an appropriate comment regarding the likely site of origin of the tumour. CGIN is suspected in samples containing endocervical cells showing both architectural and cytological abnormality: on primary screening, identification is often made on the architectural appearance of the groups and individual cell morphology confirms the diagnosis. The architectural appearances of CGIN are characterised by cells in clusters with some nuclear overlapping, crowding, rosette formation and pseudostratified strips. There is poor cohesion of cells at the edges of the groups leading to an appearance known as feathering. The nuclear features of glandular neoplasia are similar to those of high-grade squamous dyskaryosis (Figure 9.15). The presence of necrotic debris and inflammatory cells (background diathesis) suggests invasion. However, the presence or absence of invasion in glandular neoplasia cannot reliably be assessed in either conventional cytology or LBC as the features of high-grade CGIN and early invasion overlap.

Identification of non-cervical glandular lesions is rare in samples taken for routine cervical screening, accounting for 3.3/100 000 samples in data reported from Australia. Almost all are from invasive tumours, the majority of which are endometrial in origin. The higher the grade and stage of a non-cervical tumour, the greater the likelihood that exfoliated cells will appear in a cervical sample.

Borderline nuclear changes

In a small proportion of cases, it is not possible to decide whether the nuclear changes in squamous epithelial cells can be attributed to an inflammatory response or to neoplasia. In such cases, a report of 'borderline changes' is given and the woman is kept under cytological surveillance and only referred for colposcopy if the changes persist or increase in severity. This is a common problem in specimens containing evidence of HPV infection, as the koilocytes often have slightly abnormal nuclei but the changes are not sufficient to warrant an unequivocal diagnosis of mild dyskaryosis (Figure 9.11). Similarly, endocervical cells showing equivocal changes are reported as borderline but in this case the woman is referred immediately for colposcopy because there is evidence from case series that women with borderline changes in endocervical cells have increased rates of malignant and preinvasive disease.

MANAGEMENT OF ABNORMAL CERVICAL CYTOLOGY

The management of women with specimens showing moderate or severe dyskaryosis or features suggestive of squamous dyskaryosis is well defined but the management of women with mild dyskaryosis is controversial. The main aim of management is to ensure that all women with an abnormal test result receive appropriate treatment and follow-up. It is important to ensure that facilities are available for this and expert colposcopic opinion can be provided without delay. Guidance from the NHSCSP, based on professional consensus and published evidence, is summarised in Table 9.2.

FOLLOW-UP AFTER COLPOSCOPY AND TREATMENT

The duration and frequency of cytological follow-up after colposcopy depends on the grade of the lesion identified and the treatment given and is guided by the knowledge of a persistent risk of cervical cancer for at least 10 years and possibly longer after treatment for CIN, especially high grade CIN and CGIN.

Current NHSCSP guidance recommends that women treated by local excisional or ablative methods for high-grade disease (CIN2, CIN3 or CGIN) require 6- and 12-month follow-up cytology and annual cytology for the subsequent 9 years at least, before returning to routine screening. Women similarly treated for low-grade disease (HPV change only or CIN1) require 6-, 12- and 24-month follow-up cytology and, if all results are negative, they may be returned to routine screening.

Women referred with high-grade cytological abnormality in which colposcopy and biopsy fail to demonstrate a high-grade lesion should be closely followed-up by colposcopy and cytology and if high-grade cytological abnormality persists, excisional treatment is recommended.

Women referred with low-grade cytological abnormality (mild dyskaryosis or borderline change) who are found to have a low-grade lesion may be treated or followed up at 6-monthly intervals in the colposcopy clinic.

Women referred with low-grade cytological abnormality who have a satisfactory normal colposcopic examination should have a repeat cytological assessment 6 months after the referral sample and management should be determined by the result of that sample: if normal, returned to routine screening; if borderline, a repeat cytology test at 12 months; if mild dyskaryosis, colposcopy with a repeat cytology test in 12 months; any other result warrants immediate repeat colposcopy.

Vaginal-vault cytology tests are valuable in the follow-up of women who have had CIN managed by hysterectomy rather than by local treatment. Although hysterectomy is often the treatment of choice in cases of invasive cervical cancer, it is rarely indicated for the treatment of CIN. It has a place, however, following local excisional treatment where histological examination of the excision margins indicates incomplete removal of CIN or where follow-up cytology indicates residual or recurrent intraepithelial neoplasia: such women are at risk not only of cervical but also of vaginal invasive disease. For women with completely excised CIN at hysterectomy, cytological follow-up should be performed at 6 and 18 months after surgery and, if both are normal, no further cytological follow-up is required. For women with incomplete or uncertain excision of CIN at hysterectomy, follow-up should be performed as if the cervix were still in situ (see above).

Vault cytology tests after hysterectomy for invasive cervical cancer are often difficult to interpret microscopically, as reparative or radiotherapy changes, granulation tissue or even prolapsed fallopian tube tissue, can mimic neoplasia. They offer no lead time advantage in the diagnosis of recurrent invasive disease and consequently are not now recommended in many gynaecological oncology units.

The future of cervical cytology

There is no doubt that a well-organised cervical screening programme is an effective method of reducing mortality and morbidity from cervical cancer. However, the programme is costly and, in countries without a nationally funded programme, it is the women least at risk who can afford a regular cytology test. Moreover, there is a high false-negative rate associated with the Papanicolaou test, due in part to poor sampling technique but also to errors of reporting. The challenge, therefore, is to develop a more cost-effective and more accurate method of screening. Three new approaches to screening are being implemented or are under investigation, namely LBC, automated analysis of cervical samples and testing for HPV infection.

Liquid-based cytology

In this technique, the resulting slide preparations consist of a near monolayer of epithelial cells largely unobscured by blood, inflammatory cells or mucus. As a result, the number of specimens reported as inadequate falls dramatically and the preparations are easier to interpret, resulting in increased laboratory productivity. Studies in the UK, USA and elsewhere have clearly demonstrated a marked reduction in the inadequate specimen rate and increased productivity with no loss of sensitivity. Many laboratories in the USA have fully converted to LBC and the NHSCSP has fully converted to LBC from the end of 2008. Furthermore, the near monolayer preparations are ideal for computer aided analysis and the residual cellular material in the specimen vial may be used for HPV and other emerging molecular testing.

Automated analysis of cervical cytology tests

There have been several occasions recently both in the UK and the USA when laboratories have been severely criticised by the press and public for failing to provide a reliable cytodiagnostic service. Errors of reporting cervical cytology tests have put women's lives at risk and have led to loss of confidence in the cervical screening programme. The response to this unfortunate situation has been to examine alternative methods of screening which might offer a higher degree of accuracy and reliability of performance.

One method which is currently under intense investigation is the automated analysis of cervical cytology tests. A model automated system should meet the following specifications:

- The system should detect all samples that contain neoplastic cells (high sensitivity).

- The system should not flag 'false alarms' on normal cells (high specificity).

- The system should not render the cytology test unsuitable for classical microscopic review.

- The results should be reproducible.

- The system should identify inadequate cytology tests.

- The system should operate cost effectively.

Such systems are currently under evaluation in the UK with a view to their introduction in the NHSCSP. It is worth noting that they can function almost continuously and to achieve cost-effective utilisation, some laboratory reconfiguration will almost certainly be necessary.

HPV testing

Within the last 20 years, evidence has accumulated which indicates that HPV plays a pivotal role in the development of most cervical cancers. The evidence is drawn from studies of the prevalence of DNA sequences from oncogenic HPV strains (notably types 16 and 18) in cancerous and precancerous cervical lesions and from demonstration of the transforming properties of these cancer-associated HPV types in vitro and in experimental animals. Moreover, while it is recognised that many sexually active women become infected with HPV, prospective studies have shown that women with persisting oncogenic HPV infection in the cervical epithelium have a much greater risk of developing CIN3 and invasive carcinoma (odds ratio of 100-fold or more) than women who are HPV-negative. These observations have led to the suggestion that testing for oncogenic types of HPV could be used in a number of ways to refine existing screening programmes:

- increase the specificity of the cytology test
- triage of low-grade cytology tests
- follow-up after treatment
- primary screening.

Since HPV infection is common in sexually active young women, persisting infection with oncogenic types of HPV is the principal risk factor for development of CIN and HPV is always present in preceding cervical samples from women who develop cervical cancer; the negative predictive value of a negative test for oncogenic HPV types is very high. Women over the age of 30 years of age with a negative HPV test are at virtually zero risk of developing cervical cancer in the decade following the negative test. It has been suggested, therefore, that the screening interval could be increased in women over 30 years who are both HPV and cytology-negative and screening could be ceased in women over 50 years with a negative cytology screening history who are HPV and cytology negative at age 50 years.

It is well recognised that a proportion of women with low-grade cytological abnormality will in fact have concurrent high-grade CIN and a number of studies have assessed the accuracy of HPV testing to triage women with a test showing borderline change or mild dyskaryosis to colposcopy rather than repeat cytology testing. Recent meta-analysis has shown that HPV testing is more accurate (higher sensitivity and similar specificity) than cytology in triage of women with borderline nuclear changes. However, HPV testing does not show significantly higher sensitivity and has significantly lower specificity than repeat cytology in triage of women with mild dyskaryosis.

Recurrent or residual disease will be found in about 10% of women within 2 years after treatment for CIN and the risk of recurrence is higher in women older than 50 years. The identification of an indicator to predict successful treatment and allow shortening of the follow-up period would be very valuable. A recent meta-analysis has shown that HPV testing identifies residual disease earlier and with higher sensitivity and similar specificity to follow-up cytology or histological assessment of resection margins. There are, however, as yet insufficient long-term data to formulate detailed evidence based follow-up algorithms.

While it is recognised that cervical cytological screening has significantly reduced the incidence of and mortality from cervical cancer, recently the sensitivity and specificity of the test have been questioned and false-negative tests in particular highlighted by well-publicised failures of screening programmes. There is pressure to develop an alternative screening test for cervical cancer prevention and the role of HPV testing as the primary screening test, with or without secondary triage by cytology, has been extensively explored. A systematic review and meta-analysis of studies comparing primary HPV testing to cytology with regard to their accuracy in detection of high-grade CIN have shown that HPV testing is more sensitive than cytology but less specific. The combination of HPV testing and cytology has the highest sensitivity but lowest specificity. However, reduction of the incidence of or mortality from cervical cancer among HPV-screened women compared with cytologically screened women has not been demonstrated and the results of further studies are awaited.

Other gynaecological cytology

Cytology can also contribute to the evaluation of functional and neoplastic lesions of the female genital tract other than in the cervix in a number of scenarios.

SEROUS FLUID

Accumulation of serous fluid in the abdominal cavity (ascites) may be the presenting feature of malignant disease and, in adult females, peritoneal involvement is most often seen with ovarian carcinoma, followed by breast and gastrointestinal carcinoma and malignant lymphoma. Morphological and immunocytochemical studies of ascitic fluid obtained by transabdominal needle aspiration in a woman with a

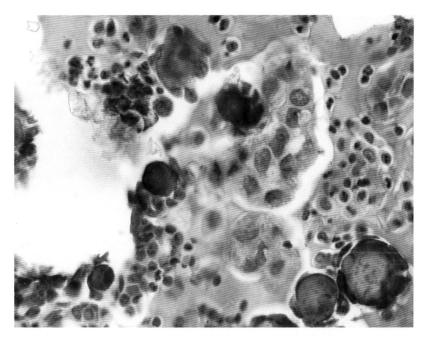

Figure 9.17. Papillary serous carcinoma in ascitic fluid: papillary groups of vacuolated malignant epithelial cells associated with psammoma bodies

suspected ovarian, tubal or primary peritoneal malignancy may allow confirmation of the diagnosis (Figure 9.17) or if the primary site is not already established may indicate the primary site or narrow the differential. Immunocytochemistry is particularly useful to distinguish between adenocarcinoma, mesothelioma and reactive mesothelial proliferation and differential expression of cytokeratins 7 and 20, carcinoembryonic antigen and CA125 can be used to distinguish ovarian, tubal and primary peritoneal adenocarcinoma from gastrointestinal adenocarcinoma and adenocarcinoma from other sites.

Cytological examination of peritoneal washings obtained at the time of surgery for ovarian, tubal or endometrial carcinoma is an established part of the FIGO staging. The finding of malignant cells in peritoneal washings is an important variable that predicts a poor prognosis at all stages of ovarian carcinoma. However, in endometrial carcinoma positive peritoneal washing cytology is related to advanced-stage disease and other adverse prognostic factors such as high-grade tumour and vascular space involvement and it is uncertain if positive peritoneal washing cytology is an independent adverse prognostic factor in stage I disease.

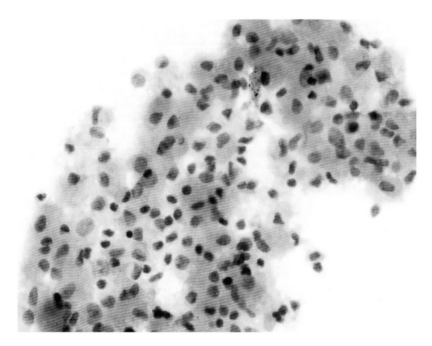

Figure 9.18. Aspirate from a luteal cyst of the ovary: small uniform granulosa cells are admixed with large luteinised cells characterised by abundant finely vacuolated pink cytoplasm

FINE-NEEDLE ASPIRATION CYTOLOGY

Fine-needle aspiration of ovarian lesions can be valuable as a diagnostic or therapeutic procedure. Ovarian lesions can be aspirated via the vagina or rectum, transabdominally, or at laparoscopy or laparotomy. Ultrasound-guided transvaginal aspiration is the preferred method in many units. Morphological evaluation combined with immunocytochemistry and evaluation of the clinical and radiological features permits distinction of functional from neoplastic cysts and the distinction of primary epithelial, sex-cord stromal, germ cell and metastatic tumours (Figure 9.18).

Reference

1.   British Society for Clinical Cytology. *Taking Cervical Smears*. London: BSCC; [www.clinicalcytology.co.uk/resources/video/video.pdf?order=true].

Further reading

Arbyn M, Sasieni P, Meijer CJLM, Clavel C, Koliopoulos G, Dillner J. Clinical applications of HPV testing: a summary of recent meta-analyses. *Vaccine* 2006;24(S3):78–89.

Buckley CH, Fox H. *Biopsy Pathology of the Endometrium*. London: Arnold; 2002.

Denton K, Herbert A, Turnbull LA, Waddell CA, Desai M, Rana D, *et al*. The revised BSCC terminology for cervical cytology 2007. *Cytopathology* 2008;19:137–57.

Evans DMD, Hudson EA, Brown CL, Boddington MM, Hughes HE, MacKenzie EFD, *et al*. Terminology in gynaecological cytopathology: report of the working party of the BSCC. *J Clin Pathol* 1986;39:933–44.

Fox H, Sebire NJ. *Pathology of the Placenta*. 3rd ed. London: Saunders; 2007.

Fox H, Wells M, editors. *Haines & Taylor Obstetrical and Gynaecological Pathology*. Edinburgh: Churchill Livingstone; 2003.

Luesley D, Leeson S, editors. *Colposcopy and Programme Management*. NHSCSP Publication 20. Sheffield: NHSCSP; 2004.

Solomon D, Nayar R. *The Bethesda System for Reporting Cervical Cytology: Definitions, Criteria and Explanatory Notes*. 2nd ed. New York: Springer; 2004.

Tavassoli FA, Devilee P, editors. *Tumours of the Breast and Female Genital Organs, World Health Organization Classification of Tumours*. Lyon: IARC Press; 2003. p. 113–432.

Index

stromal nodule, endometrium 95

stromal sarcoma

    cervix 62

    endometrium 94

strumal carcinoid tumour of ovary 166, 168

struma ovarii 166, 167

SurePath™ 207

    see also liquid-based cytology

syphilis 7, 27, 41, 194

tamoxifen 71–2, 78, 80

teratomas 161, 164–6, 169

    immature 164, 165, 166

    malignant change 164, 166

    mature cystic 118, 164–6

    monophyletic 164, 166

    ruptured mature cystic 122, 123, 164–6

theca–lutein cysts 125–9

thecomas of ovary 153–6

ThinPrep® 207

    see also liquid-based cytology

toxoplasmosis 194

transformation zone 35, 36, 203

transitional cell carcinoma of ovary 141–4

Trichomonas vaginalis, cervical cytology 208, 211

trichomoniasis 27, 42

triploidy 183–4

trophoblast, extravillous 192–3

trophoblastic disease

    gestational 179–87

    persistent 183, 184, 185

trophoblastic tumour

    epithelioid 187

    placental site 186–7, 188

tuberculosis

    endometrial 76, 78

    fallopian tube 112–14

tubo-ovarian abscess 110

twin pregnancy, placenta in 197–9

twin-to-twin transfusion syndrome 197–9

urethral carcinoma 24

uterine sarcoma, undifferentiated 94

uteroplacental vessels 192–3

vagina 26–34

    infections 26–7

    inflammation 26–7

    neoplasms 29–32

vaginal adenosis 27–8, 32, 33

vaginal carcinoma 29–32

    clear-cell adenocarcinoma 30–1

    metastatic 29, 30

    other adenocarcinomas 32, 33

    squamous cell 29–30

vaginal intraepithelial neoplasia (VAIN) 28–9

vaginal-vault cytology 223

vasculitis, myometrium 99

verrucous carcinoma, vulva 20–1

villitis 194

VIN *see* vulval intraepithelial neoplasia

viral infections, cervix 40–1

virilisation 129, 130, 132, 157

vulva 1–25

    benign tumours 16–17

    dermatological disorders 1–3

    inflammation 5–10

    malignant tumours 17–24

    non-invasive, intraepithelial neoplastic lesions 10–14

    non-neoplastic cysts 14–16

    pigmented lesions 11, 13, 21–2

vulval carcinoma 2, 17–21

    invasive squamous cell 17–19

    metastatic 24, 25

    microinvasive squamous cell 20, 21

    staging system 19, 20

    verrucous 20–1

    VIN and 13–14, 19

vulval dystrophies 1

vulval intraepithelial neoplasia (VIN) 10–14, 19

    basaloid 11, 12

    Bowenoid (warty) 11, 12

    differentiated 11

    grading 11, 13

    undifferentiated 11, 12, 13

vulvitis

    infective 5–10

    non-infective 5

Walthard's rest, cystic 115, 117

warts, genital 8–10, 43–5

yolk sac tumours 162, 163